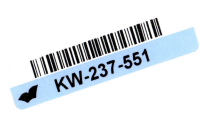

ORAL HEALTH

ORAL HEALTH
Diet and other factors

The Report of the British Nutrition Foundation's Task Force

Edited by Ursula Arens
(British Nutrition Foundation)

**Published by Elsevier
for the British Nutrition Foundation**

ELSEVIER

Amsterdam - Lausanne - New York - Oxford - Shannon - Singapore - Tokyo

ELSEVIER SCIENCE B.V.
Sara Burgerhartstraat 25
P.O. Box 211, 1000 AE Amsterdam, The Netherlands

Library of Congress Cataloging in Publication Data

```
Oral health--diet and other factors : the report of the British
  Nutrition Foundation's Task Force / edited by Ursula Arens.
       p.   cm.
    "Published by Elsevier for the British Nutrition Foundation."
    Includes bibliographical references and index.
    ISBN 0-444-50025-1
    1. Mouth--Diseases--Nutritional aspects. 2. Teeth--Diseases-
  -Nutritional aspects.   I. Arens, Ursula. II. British Nutrition
  Foundation.  Oral Health Task Force.
  RK305.068  1998
  617.6'01--dc21                              98-39770
                                                 CIP
```

ISBN: 0-444-50025-1

⊚ The paper used in this publication meets the requirements of ANSI/NISO Z39.48-1992 (Permanence of Paper).
Printed in The Netherlands.

CONTENTS

MEMBERSHIP OF THE BNF ORAL HEALTH

TASK FORCE

Chairman
Jack Edelman
Honorary Vice President
British Nutrition Foundation

Members
Raman Bedi
Professor of Transcultural
Oral Health
Centre for Transcultural Oral
Health
Eastman Dental Institute for
Oral Health Care Sciences
256 Grays Inn Road
London WC1X 8LD

David Beighton
Professor of Oral
Microbiology
Department of Oral
Microbiology
Guy's, King's and St Thomas'
School of Dentistry
Caldecot Road
London SE5 9RW

Nino M Binns
Nutrition Manager
Coca-Cola Greater Europe
1 Queen Caroline Street
London W6 9HQ
Visiting Professor in
Nutrition, University of Ulster
at Coleraine

Sally Craig
Lecturer in Child Dental
Health
Department of Child Dental
Health
School of Clinical Dentistry
Claremont Crescent
Sheffield S10 2TA
(appointed in association with
the British Dental
Association)

Martin C Downer
Honorary Professor
Centre for Transcultural Oral
Health
Eastman Dental Institute for
Oral Health Care Sciences
256 Grays Inn Road
London WC1X 8LD

W Michael Edgar
Emeritus Professor of Dental
Sciences
Oral Biology Unit
School of Dentistry
University of Liverpool
Liverpool L69 3BX

Catherine Geissler
Professor of Nutrition
Head of Division of Health
Sciences
King's College
Campden Hill Road
London W8 7AH

Phillip J Holloway
Emeritus Professor of Child
Dental Health
Dental Health Unit
Unit 3a, Skelton House
Manchester Science Park
Lloyd St North
Manchester M15 6SH

David Wray
Professor of Oral Medicine
Glasgow Dental School
378 Sauchiehall Street
Glasgow G2 3JZ
(Appointed in association
with the Royal College of
Surgeons, Faculty of Dental
Surgery)

Observers
Anthony Hawkes
Senior Dental Officer
Department of Health
Office of Chief Dental Officer
(Room 319)
Richmond House
79 Whitehall
London SW1A 2NS

Martin Wiseman
Head of Nutrition Unit
Department of Health
Nutrition Unit (Room 632B)
Skipton House
80 London Road
London SE1 6LW
Visiting Professor in
Nutrition, University of
Southampton

Corresponding members
William H Bowen
Welcher Professor of Dental
Research
Rochester Caries Research
Center
601 Elmwood Avenue
New York 14642
USA

Denis O'Mullane
Professor of Preventive and
Paediatric Dentistry
Director of Oral Health
Services Research Centre
University Dental School and
Hospital
University College Cork
Wilton, Cork
Ireland

Brian Wharton
Director-General (until
October 1997)
British Nutrition Foundation

Ursula Arens
Senior Nutrition Scientist
British Nutrition Foundation
(Secretary to the Task Force
until November 1996; Editor
of the Task Force Report)

Laura Ellis (now Mrs Laura
Hanley)
Nutrition Scientist
British Nutrition Foundation
(Secretary to the Task Force
from December 1996 until
August 1997)

Elisa Pons
PA to the Science Group
British Nutrition Foundation

TERMS OF REFERENCE

The Task Force was invited by the Council of the British Nutrition Foundation to:

1 Review the relationship of nutrition and diet (and where necessary other factors) to oral health.

2 Prepare a report and, should it see fit, draw conclusions, make recommendations and identify areas for future research.

This Report is the collective work of all the members of the Task Force. Authors of the first draft of each chapter are given below.

1   Structures of the mouth
    Professor WM Edgar
2   The oral microflora
    Professor D Beighton
3   Food components relevant to oral health
    Professor C Geissler
4   Dental caries—aetiology and pathogenesis
    Professors D Beighton and WM Edgar
5   Dental caries—epidemiology in the UK
    Professors MC Downer, R Bedi and PJ Holloway
6   Dental caries—diet and nutrition
    Professor PJ Holloway
7   Tooth wear
    Professor WM Edgar
8   Enamel defects
    Professor NM Binns and Mrs S Craig
9   Periodontal diseases
    Professor WM Edgar
10 Oral cancer
    Professors MC Downer, R Bedi and D Wray
11 Oral soft tissue and salivary gland disease
    Professor D Wray
12 The fetus
    Professor BA Wharton
13 Infants and children
    Mrs S Craig
14 Older people
    *Professors D Wray and A Walls**
15 People living in areas of multiple deprivation
    Professors Bedi and PJ Holloway
16 Culture and diet
    Professor R Bedi
17 Ill-health and disease
    Professor D Wray

* Guest author.

ACKNOWLEDGEMENTS

The Task Force gratefully acknowledges the help received from Professor Crispian Scully (Eastman Dental Institute for Oral Health Care Sciences) and Professor Angus Walls (Department of Restorative Dentistry, University of Newcastle) in the drafting of some sections of the report.

PREFACE

The British Nutrition Foundation organises independent 'Task Forces' to review, analyse and report in depth upon specific areas of interest and importance in the field of human nutrition. These expert committees consist of acknowledged specialists, and operate completely independently of the Foundation. The Oral Health Task Force has reviewed and discussed much published information. This report presents the deliberations and findings of the Task Force and gives its conclusions and recommendations.

There is little need to stress the importance of oral disease in the population. The personal experience of almost everyone reading this account testifies to that. Although national mortality figures are low, other statistics relating to oral disease are substantial despite the remarkable improvement in the nation's oral health over the last quarter century; before then the problem of dental caries was essentially out of control.

There has been a variety of conferences, workshops and reports on oral health in recent years, but the Council of the BNF decided that the subject is still of sufficient interest and importance to individuals, health professionals, industry and the authorities responsible for the nation's health for this Task Force to be convened.

Pain, disfigurement, embarrassment and reduction in the quality of life are difficult to measure but are widespread because of oral health problems. Despite the recent improvement, which appears, however, to be levelling off, large numbers of children still suffer anxiety and discomfort in the dentist's chair. One of the most upsetting aspects of dentistry, admitted by the adult population, is that associated with tooth extraction, experienced as a child. Even now, by the age of 15 years most children have had at least one decayed tooth filled, and toothache is still all too common among adults as well as children. Many of the problems worsen with age and older people frequently have difficulties with eating and dental pain, and also with social relationships because of embarrassment about some aspect of their dentition.

In Britain, close on £2 billion is spent on dental treatment each year and to this must be added the time lost at work or school. A disease still as prevalent as this must continue to command attention. This Report also covers diseases of the mouth, some of which are considerably less widespread but, in some cases, more life-threatening.

Many of the problems can be alleviated by changes in personal habits—oral hygiene, diet, smoking and alcohol consumption. That is easy to say, of course, but difficult to achieve. Unfortunately, as with many other health problems, it is socially disadvantaged people that suffer most from oral disease, and some ethnic groups are also more prone than the general population. So, targeting is as important as in most health issues, and this often comes up against financial worries or cultural resistance to change, as well as ignorance, or even fear, of scientific developments.

This Report analyses and discusses available scientific evidence and seeks to support measures needed to alleviate the widespread incidence of oral disease. The agreed opinions expressed are entirely those of the membership of the Task Force.

I am most grateful to the members of the Task Force who have contributed their time and expertise so generously, and to others who have helped with advice and comment. My sincere thanks also go to the Secretariat at the Foundation for their excellent support.

Jack Edelman
Chairman of the Task Force

1

STRUCTURES OF THE MOUTH

1.1 TEETH

The teeth and their supporting structures possess many features which are unique, as well as some which are more widespread among the tissues of the body. A general description of the teeth, their formation, chemical and physical nature, and their micro- and macroscopic structure is given here to highlight aspects which may be unfamiliar to those without specialist knowledge of the dentition.

1.1.1 Tooth anatomy

A schematic cross-section of a tooth in its bony socket is shown in Figure 1.1. The tooth is composed mainly of a bone-like substance, *dentine*,

which is covered by a layer of hard *enamel* which helps the tooth to resist being worn away by attrition due to decades of chewing. The third hard tissue—*cementum*—covers the *root* of the tooth and attaches it to the surrounding *alveolar bone* by means of the strong collagen fibres of the *periodontal ligament*. These tissues—cementum, alveolar bone and periodontal ligament—can be considered as a unit, the *periodontium*. Above the bony socket, the gum or *gingiva* is covered by a mucous membrane, and between the enamel and the gingiva is a crevice called the *gingival crevice* or *sulcus*. At the base of the crevice is the *epithelial attachment* of the soft tissues to the enamel. With age and disease, this attachment migrates down to the root to expose cementum and/or dentine. The *anatomical crown* of the tooth is that part covered by

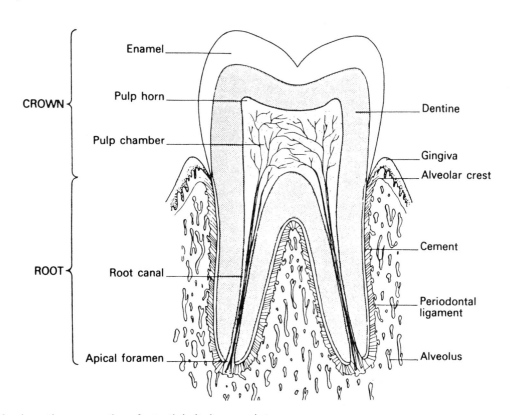

Figure 1.1 A schematic cross-section of a tooth in its bony socket.
Source: Osborn (1981).

the enamel; the *clinical crown* is defined as that part of the tooth which is above the gum margin, whether or not it is covered by enamel. Inside the dentine is the *pulp cavity* containing the *dental pulp*, a fibrous tissue with a few blood vessels and nerves which maintains the vitality (and sensitivity) of the dentine. The pulp is connected by the *root canal* to the tissues at the *apex of the root*; because of its narrowness, the blood vessels to the pulp can easily be occluded with resulting death or *necrosis* of the pulp.

In primates, including man, the teeth erupt to form two *dentitions* (Table 1.1). The *primary* or *deciduous* dentition (milk teeth) which starts to erupt at about six months and is usually complete by three years of age, and the *secondary* or permanent dentition starting with the first permanent molar teeth at around six years and ending with the third molars (wisdom teeth) erupting at 18–25 years.

The names of the teeth reflect their function during mastication:

- *incisors*   cutting
- *canines*   stabbing, tearing
- *premolars*   grinding
- *molars*   crushing

The deciduous teeth are normally 20 in number—four incisors, two canines and four molars in each jaw (upper, *maxilla*; lower, *mandibular*) (Figure 1.2). These are replaced in the growing child by the larger permanent teeth which normally total 32—four incisors, two canines, four premolars and six molars in each jaw. Between the age of six years, with the eruption of the first permanent molar, and approximately 12 years, when the last deciduous tooth is replaced by its permanent successor, the child is said to be in the mixed dentition stage.

1.1.2 Tooth formation

In the earliest stages of its development, the embryo is made up of two types of cells, the endodermal cells which eventually make up the alimentary and respiratory systems, and the ectodermal cells which form external and lining cells such as skin, mucous membranes, and the nervous system. Also derived from the primitive ectoderm are the mesodermal cells, which eventually give rise to the circulatory system and most of the muscles and connective tissues of the body, including the bones. The process by which these primitive cell-types become specialised is known as *differentiation*. The control of differentiation is a highly complex process right at the heart of biological knowledge. However,

Table 1.1 Chronology of tooth development

	Tooth	Tooth germ fully formed	Dentine formation begins	Crown formation complete	Eruption	Root complete
Deciduous	Incisors	3–4 months fetal life	4–6 months fetal life	2–3 months	6–9 months	1–1½ years after eruption
	Canines			9 months	16–18 months	
	1st molars			6 months	12–14 months	
	2nd molars			12 months	20–30 months	
	Incisors	30th week fetal life	3–4 months (upper lateral incisor 10–12 months)	4–5 years	Lower 6–8 years Upper 7–9 years	2–3 years after eruption
	Canines	30th week fetal life	4–5 months	6–7 years	Lower 9–10 years Upper 11–12 years	
	Premolars	30th week fetal life	1½–2½ years	5–7 years	10–12 years	
	1st molars	24th week fetal life	Birth	2½–3 years	6–7 years	
	2nd molars	6th month	2½–3 years	7–8 years	11–13 years	
	3rd molars	6th year	7–10 years	12–16 years	17–21 years	

Source: Scott and Symons (1985). Reprinted with permission of Churchill Livingstone.

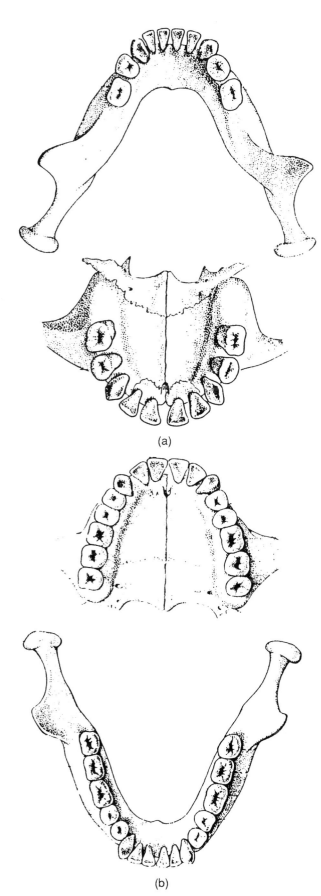

(a)

(b)

Figure 1.2 Upper and lower jaws of child (a) and adult (b).
Source: Frick *et al.* (1990). Reproduced with permission: S. Karger AG, Basel.

one facet of significance is the process of *induction*—in order to differentiate into the right type of tissue, a cell may be induced by adjacent cells to form, for example, a sweat gland, a hair follicle or a tooth. Induction requires the interaction between cells of different embryonic origin, particularly, those of ectodermal and mesodermal origin, known as *epithelial* and *mesenchymal* cells, respectively.

At about the sixth week of embryonic life, the precursors of the oral cavity consist of maxillary and mandibular processes of mesenchyme covered by epithelium. The beginning of tooth formation is marked by a thickening of the epithelium, which, with time, begins to grow down into the underlying mesenchyme in each jaw. Part of this *epithelial band* forms a fold which is the beginning of the separation of the lips and cheeks from the gums, and the remainder forms the *dental lamina* from which the teeth develop. Shortly after its initiation, the dental lamina begins to form swellings called enamel organs which mark out the future teeth—first the deciduous teeth, and beginning at about 16 weeks of embryonic life, the future permanent teeth. The enamel organs forming the second and third permanent molars begin to appear after birth.

At first, the enamel organ is a simple ball of epithelial cells with a surrounding condensation of mesenchyme, but it soon begins to form a cap-shaped and then a bell-shaped structure which, together with its associated mesenchyme, is known as the *tooth germ*. Inside the bell of epithelium, the mesenchyme (*dental papilla*) will become the dental pulp, while that outside (the *dental follicle*) will form a capsule to control the size of the bony cavity in which the developing tooth is situated. The shape of the future crown will be determined by the relative rate of growth of epithelium and mesenchyme.

At this point, the formation of the enamel and dentine is initiated by the epithelium, which induces the differentiation of dentine-forming cells (*odontoblasts*) in the dental papilla. As soon as dentine formation commences, there follows the induction of the epithelial cells to produce enamel-forming cells (*ameloblasts*).

1.1.3 Enamel

The first enamel secreted by the ameloblasts consists of a soft material containing approximately 30% of mineral crystals and 20% of protein material. The function of the latter is to define the space which the enamel will occupy when mature, and perhaps to assist in the formation and orientation of the crystals.

As the enamel layer reaches its full thickness, however, further changes occur which collectively are known as *enamel maturation*. There is a loss of protein, accompanied by a large increase in mineral content, so that the final mature enamel is made up of 95% mineral and only 1% protein. This high mineral content is needed for the hardness of enamel, and is achieved by the removal of protein. In the other mineralised tissues (bone, dentine, cementum), the protein in which the mineral is laid down is not removed, resulting in a maximum mineral content of 70%.

The mineral is an almost insoluble calcium phosphate having many of the characteristics of a form of rock known as *hydroxyapatite*. Its basic formula is:

$$Ca_{10}(PO_4)_6(OH)_2$$

In biological tissues, some of the ions are missing and/or substituted by others, e.g. CO_3^{2-} ions may replace PO_4^{3-} ions. The most important substitution is that of F^- for OH^-, which results in a crystal which is more stable ('stronger') and, thus, more able to resist attack during the caries process.

The crystals, unlike those in the other hard tissues, are much larger (about 1000 nm long, 40 nm wide and 10 nm thick), and are oriented during secretion and growth by the ameloblasts. Their orientation leads to the formation of structural units known as enamel *rods* or *prisms*, about 3–6 μm in diameter which, because of the change in crystal orientation at their periphery, form 'fault lines' along which acids can diffuse and cracks can propagate. Thus enamel is also brittle, as well as being hard. Its porosity is very low, and although to a limited extent it is permeable, this is only to water and other small molecules. Its surface activity is high and this encourages the attachment of proteins and bacteria from saliva to form *pellicle* and *plaque*. Enamel is translucent but if subjected to acid attack it becomes opaque due to the increased porosity. As the enamel becomes thin with increasing age due to tooth wear, the underlying dentine, which is greyish-yellow, shows through. Attempts to make the teeth look white again by use of an abrasive toothpaste merely make the problem worse.

Tooth wear is a normal feature of ageing, and is due to a combination of the effects of attrition (masticatory grinding forces), abrasion (from foods or toothpaste etc) and erosion (softening of enamel by acid).

1.1.4 Dentine

Young odontoblasts immediately after differentiation have more than one short finger-like extension pointing towards the junction between future dentine and future enamel, but soon the small fingers unite to form a single *odontoblast process*. The first secretion consists of a protein *matrix* containing collagen fibres within a proteoglycan ground substance, together with *matrix vesicles*, which have been implicated in the formation of mineral crystals. In dentine nearest to the enamel (or cementum), many of the fibres are arranged perpendicular to the enamel-dentine junction but, in the bulk of dentine, the predominant fibre direction is perpendicular to the odontoblast process, and matrix vesicles are absent. As dentine is laid down, the odontoblasts move away from the dentine-enamel junction, and each odontoblast process is left behind within a *tubule*.

Shortly after being formed by the odontoblast, the dentine matrix becomes mineralised by the formation of hydroxyapatite crystals. These are smaller than in enamel (about 100 nm long and 2–4 nm thick), and are often aligned parallel to the collagen fibres. However, in dentine there are regions known as calcospherites in which some of the crystals are oriented radially from a central point. The change from unmineralised predentine to mineralised dentine is controlled by the odontoblast—perhaps by secreting special proteins and/or proteoglycans, which together with collagen form a template on which apatite crystals can grow. The odontoblast is also responsible for transporting calcium and phosphate ions for mineralisation.

Mature dentine contains approximately 20% of organic material (most of which is collagen fibres), 10% of water and 70% of mineral, mainly hydroxapatite.

If dentine is exposed by loss of the enamel covering through caries or other processes, or by gum recession and subsequent removal of the cementum, it may become acutely sensitive to stimuli such as hot or cold food. The basis of this sensitivity is generally attributed to the flow of fluid within the odontoblast tubules, causing movement of the odontoblasts which is transmitted to nerves within the pulp. Nerve fibres from the pulp enter the dentine alongside the odontoblasts, but they do not penetrate far, and there are too few to explain dentinal sensitivity.

Dentine formation persists slowly throughout life (*secondary dentine*), but if the dentine becomes exposed and irritants pass down the tubules, the odontoblasts respond by first sealing off the tubules, then forming *tertiary dentine*, which is rapidly mobilised to provide a defence against possible damage to the pulp and, hence, the viability of the tooth.

With increasing age, the dentinal tubules beginning in the root become filled with mineral deposits and with degradation products of the odontoblast processes, so that the dentine is eventually impermeable and looks translucent. The process may eventually reach the dentine in the crown of the tooth. As the pulp chamber becomes filled with secondary dentine, it becomes less vital and more fibrous, and may begin to mineralise itself.

1.1.5 Periodontium—cementum

After crown formation, the epithelium of the enamel organ continues to proliferate and forms a cuff (the *epithelial root sheath*), which defines the future dentine of the root by induction of odontoblasts from cells of the dental papilla. Meanwhile, the inner layer of the mesenchymal cells of the dental follicle differentiate to form *cementoblasts*, and migrate between the epithelial cells of the root sheath to reach the predentine being laid down by the root odontoblasts. Here, the cementoblasts begin to lay down precementum, which then mineralises, incorporating collagen fibres originating from the periodontal ligament. The organic content of cementum is slightly higher than that of dentine, and at about 30%, the mineral content is proportionately reduced.

Around the neck of the tooth and in the midroot area the cementum is acellular, but at the root apex, the cementum contains cells called *cementocytes*. Cementum can be reabsorbed (e.g. during the shedding of deciduous teeth), but is less susceptible than alveolar bone. Hence, when the tooth is moved in the course of orthodonic treatment, it is the bone, not the root, which is removed to make way. In older individuals, cementum deposition often continues at the root apex, effectively lengthening the tooth (*hypercementosis*). The *periodontal ligament* extends from the alveolar bone to the cementum, and also in health extends between adjacent teeth. The surfaces of the tooth and gingivae are washed by saliva and protected by the secretory IgA system present in saliva. The gingival crevice, however, is protected by the *systemic immune system* derived from the blood, and *IgG* predominates in the gingival crevice and the *crevicular fluid* which exudes from the crevice.

1.2 SALIVARY GLANDS AND SALIVA

Saliva is a complex fluid having several important functions:

- *Lubrication* of the tongue, cheeks and lips during mastication and speech;
- *Digestion* of starch due to an enzyme (amylase) present in saliva;
- *Protection* of the teeth by controlling the chemical environment to prevent dissolution, and by controlling the oral microbiological flora via antibacterial substances, both non-immunological and immunological, especially, secretory IgA.

Saliva originates mainly from three major pairs of glands: the *parotid*, *submandibular* and *sublingual* glands. In addition, numerous *minor salivary glands* are distributed around the oral mucous membranes: the floor of the mouth, tongue, lining of the cheeks, hard and soft palate and inner surface of the lips. The composition of the fluid from each type of gland is different. The parotid glands secrete a watery, mainly *serous* fluid while the sublingual and the minor salivary glands secrete a thick, mainly *mucous* fluid. The submandibular gland is intermediate, forming a mixture of serous and mucous saliva. In addition to the mixed fluid from the glands, saliva contains traces of plasma proteins and white blood cells, which can escape via the gingival crevice, numerous bacteria, and dead cells from the mucosa of the cheeks, lips and tongue. A tiny amount of saliva is also produced by special minor glands associated with the large taste papillae at the back of the tongue.

1.2.1 Secretion of saliva

Salivary glands are made up of secretory cells arranged in the form of hollow clumps called *acini*, which are connected with a *duct system* leading the saliva to the main *secretory duct* where it enters the mouth. The saliva is formed in the acini controlled by the nerves of the *autonomic nervous system*, responding mainly to reflex stimuli associated with the presence of food in the mouth—notably taste stimuli, and the movements of mastication including pressure on the tooth in its socket. Once formed, the saliva is modified in the ducts before reaching the mouth. This involves the removal of sodium chloride and secretion of bicarbonate ions. The 'two-stage' secretion means that the composition of saliva varies with the rate of secretion—the faster the secretion rate, the more rapid the passage of saliva through the ducts and, thus, the less time there is for the saliva to be modified. However, rapidly-secreted saliva contains high levels of sodium bicarbonate because this is secreted more rapidly and, therefore, the saliva is alkaline and an excellent buffer of acids from plaque.

The average flow of saliva in adults is about 600 ml per day. The rate of secretion of saliva is affected by several factors besides the reflexes associated with feeding. Salivation (at least from the major glands) almost ceases during sleep, but during the waking hours, a 'resting flow' of saliva keeps the mouth moist. If the body is dehydrated, however, this resting flow ceases, leading to the dryness of the mouth and pharynx associated with thirst. Saliva flow also ceases with strong emotional stimuli, such as fear and pain, which are part of the body's 'fright and flight' defences. On the other hand, the apparent increase in resting flow associated with the common sensation of 'mouth watering' on the anticipation of food is probably unreal, but an awareness of the saliva already present in the mouth. In man, the 'Pavlovian' conditioned response is weak or absent. However, the smell of food does lead to a direct reflex salivation.

1.1.1 Functions of saliva

Lubrication of the oral mucosa is mainly due to the mucous secretions, especially that of the minor salivary glands. In diseases of the salivary glands, the absence of lubrication causes great distress and loss of the quality of life through problems with eating and speech. The thick, slimy quality of mucous secretions is due to the presence of *mucous glycoproteins*, which are large molecules consisting of a linear protein backbone with side-chains of oligosaccharides. The large molecules entrap much water, and their long flexible side-chains become entangled with adjacent molecules, giving the viscous behaviour of the secretion.

The digestive function of saliva is due to the enzyme, *amylase*, which is secreted mainly in parotid saliva. Amylase breaks down starch molecules from food, which releases the disaccharide *maltose* together with some glucose and maltotriose. The importance of salivary amylase for digestion is doubtful as a whole—starch digestion occurs in individuals without salivary function. Once swallowed, amylase (being a protein) is inactivated by the acidity of the stomach and then broken down by proteolytic enzymes. However, there is evidence that after a large meal, the digestive juices of the stomach do not penetrate the food rapidly, and salivary amylase

may continue to break down starchy foodstuffs for long enough to make a significant contribution to their digestion.

As noted above, the protective function of saliva for the dentition is due to two effects: preventing the dissolution of the teeth, and controlling the microbial flora of the mouth. The salivary components which prevent the teeth from dissolving are *calcium phosphate* and *fluoride ions*, which inhibit dissolution and promote remineralisation, and *bicarbonate ions*, which neutralise and buffer the acids formed in dental plaque from dietary sugars. The availability of these components is increased in rapidly-secreted saliva associated with feeding.

Numerous antibacterial components are found in saliva:

- *Immumoglobulins* or antibodies which cause bacteria to aggregate;
- *Lysozyme*, an enzyme which breaks down the cell walls of certain groups of bacteria;
- *Lactoferrin*, a protein which binds iron and, thus, deprives bacteria of this essential nutrient;
- *Sialoperoxidase* and enzyme which, with the aid of hydrogen peroxide, oxidises another salivary component (thiocyanate) to form a new potent antibacterial agent (hypothiocyanite).

These antibacterial agents are clearly inactive against the majority of bacteria which have evolved to inhabit the oral cavity, but are probably vital in protecting this strategic point-of-entry to the body from more harmful pathogens. Indeed, it is known that in certain debilitated patients, lack of saliva may allow the entry of bacteria causing life-threatening infections.

1.3 ORAL SOFT TISSUES

1.3.1 Gingival epithelium

The gingiva is that part of the oral mucosa (mucous membrane) which covers the alveolar bone and the necks of the teeth. It is divided into the gingival epithelium proper—that between the oral mucosa itself and the gingival margin; the sulcal epithelium of the gingival sulcus; and the junctional epithelium, which forms a cuff attaching the gingiva to the teeth.

The gingival epithelium undergoes partial keratinisation, which acts as a barrier to diffusion. The sulcular epithelium is less keratinised, while the junctional epithelium does not keratinise at all. The differences probably arise

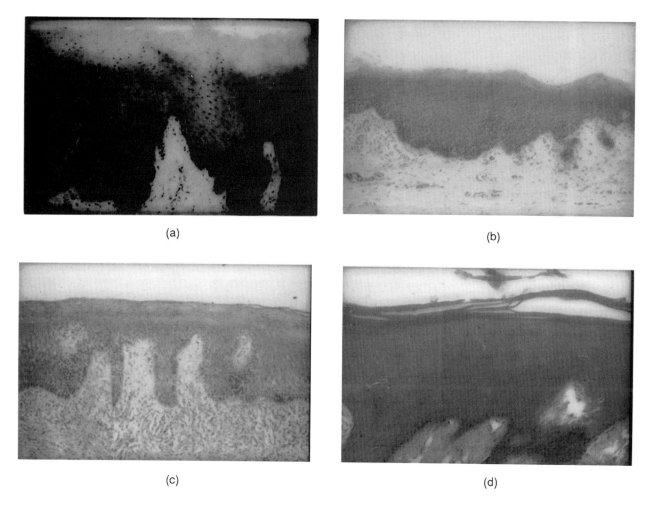

(a)

(b)

(c)

(d)

Figure 1.3 Lining mucosa.

from differences in the cells' environment rather than their genetic make-up.

1.3.2 Oral mucosa

The oral mucosa has several functions. It acts as a barrier to exogenous material, but also has an important absorption function and certain substances, such as sublingual glycerol trinitrate, that can be rapidly absorbed across the mucosa. Carcinogens, particularly in the presence of alcohol, can be rapidly absorbed across the oral mucosa.

The epithelium covering of the surface of the soft tissues of the mouth consists of stratified squamous epithelium of various kinds:

- Lining mucosa (cheeks, inner lips, floor of mouth, soft palate);
- Masticatory mucosa (hard palate, gingivae);
- Gustatory mucosa (tongue);
- Transitional mucosa (outer lips).

The inner aspects of the lips, the sulci and the cheeks are lined with mucosa which moves freely on underlying muscle, and is either non-keratinised or para-keratinised (Figure 1.3a). The mucosa covering the floor of the mouth shows similar characteristics to the lining mucosa of the lips and cheek, but tends to have minimal rete ridges (Figure 1.3b). The mucosa covering the attached gingivae, which is the area adjacent to the gum margins, comprises para-keratinising mucosa which is firmly bound to the underlying bone (Figure 1.3c). Mucoperiosteum also covers the hard palate and is ortho-keratinised (Figure 1.3d).

Masticatory mucosa is ortho-keratinised in order to withstand friction. It is firmly bound to the underlying bone forming a mucoperiosteum. Lining mucosa is thinner and redder, and moves freely on the underlying muscle. It may contain accessory (minor) mucous salivary glands for lubrication. Gustatory mucosa shows several specialised features; *filiform papillae* are pointed, slightly keratinised elevations which are valuable for moving food around the mouth; *fungiform papillae* are reddish, rounded elevations which contain taste buds; *circumvallate papillae* are larger structures surrounded by a deep circular groove, situated at the back of the mouth. They bear many taste buds within the circular groove; in the base of the groove are the ducts of small serous glands which wash the groove clear of food debris. Transitional mucosa—the red part of the outer surface of the lips— contains many blood vessels but no mucous glands. The oral mucosa, especially in the front of the mouth, is well supplied with nerves and is thus highly sensitive to external stimuli. Within the epithelium the dominant cell-type is the keratinocyte, but other cells present include antigen-presenting Langerhan's cells and melanocytes.

2

THE ORAL MICROFLORA

2.1 INTRODUCTION

The oral cavity may be colonised by over 250 different groups or taxa of microorganisms, many of which have not been completely characterised, and for which no name or method of identification has been proposed. This complexity in the composition of the oral microflora greatly hinders the comprehensive study of the microflora associated with oral health and disease. However, considerable effort has been made over many years to understand better the full complexity of the microflora of the oral cavity and of the interactions which occur between the microflora, the host and the host's diet. An appreciation of the oral microflora is essential to an understanding of oral diseases as the major oral diseases, dental caries and periodontal diseases, are the result of the interactions between the oral microflora and the tissues of the host.

2.2 PRINCIPAL MEMBERS OF THE HUMAN ORAL MICROFLORA

The principal genera present amongst the commensal (i.e. non-pathogenic) microflora of the human oral cavity are listed in Table 2.1. The predominant genera are the Streptococci, Actinomyces, Veillonella, Haemophilus, Fusobacterium and Prevotella, but the proportions of each vary on different intra-oral surfaces (Table 2.2).

2.2.1 Streptococci

The oral streptococci include *S. mutans* and *S. sobrinus* (mutans streptococci), *S. sanguis*, *S. oralis*, *S. mitis*, *S. gordonii*, *S. parasanguis*, *S. crista* (the oralis group), *S. intermedius*, *S. constellatus* and *S. anginosus* (the milleri or anginosus group) and *S. salivarius* and *S. vestibularis* (the salivarius group). The organisms originally termed 'the nutritionally variant streptococci' are now reclassified in the genus *Abi-*

Table 2.1 The principal bacterial genera isolated from the human oral cavity

	Gram positive	Gram negative
Cocci	*Enterococcus*	*Veillonella*
	Peptostreptococcus	*Neisseria*
	Streptococcus	*Bramhamella*
	Stomatococcus	
	Staphyylococcus	
Rods	*Actinomyces*	*Actinobacillus*
	Bifidobacterium	*Campylobacter*
	Rothia	*Capnocytophaga*
	Lactobacillus	*Centipeda*
	Eubacterium	*Eikenella*
	Propionibacterium	*Fusobacterium*
	Corynebacterium	*Haemophilus*
		Leptotrichia
		Porphyromonas
		Prevotella
		Selenomonas
		Simonsiella
		Treponema
		Wolinella
		'*Bacteroides*'

otrophia (Kawamura *et al.*, 1995). These bacteria may be isolated from dental plaque and saliva using selective media. They are identified in the laboratory using simple tests for the production of pre-formed enzymes and the ability to ferment specific sugars (Kilian *et al.*, 1989; Beighton *et al.*, 1991a).

Mutans streptococci are associated with the initiation and progression of dental caries. Due to their very low levels in clinical samples, techniques for their isolation involve the use of selective culture media. These bacteria are found normally in the mouth and their presence alone does not necessarily indicate the presence of active tooth decay. The ability of these bacteria to initiate tooth decay depends partly on the composition of the diet (van Palenstein Helderman *et al.*, 1996). These two species of mutans streptococci can be identified using simple tests (Beighton *et al.*, 1991b; Table 2.3). In many studies, these two species are not differentiated

Table 2.2 Distribution of commensal bacteria in the adult oral cavity

Species	Saliva	Tongue	Supra-gingival plaque	Sub-gingival plaque
Streptococcus salivaruis	+++	+++	0	0
Streptococcus sanguis	++	++	+++	+
Streptococcus oralis	++	++	++	+++
'milleri group'	±	±	+ to +++	0
Streptococcus mutans	± to +	±	+ to +++	0
Streptococcus sobrinus	0 to ±	0 to ±	0 to +	±
Lactobacillus spp.	0 to ±	+	+	++
Actinomyces spp.	++	+	+++±	± to +
Capnocytophaga spp.	0	0	±	± to +++
Treponema spp.	0	0	+	± to +++
Prevotella spp.	0 to ±	0 to ±	++	++
Veillonella alcalescens	+	+	0	0 to +++
Porphyromonas gingivalis	0	0		
Actinobacillus				
actinomycetemcomitans	0 to ±	0	±	0 to +

Key:
0 = not frequently detected.
± = rarely present.
+ = usually present in low numbers.
++ = usually present in moderate numbers.
+++ = usually present in high numbers.

Table 2.3 Scheme for the identification of *S. mutans* and *S. sobrinus*

Biochemical test	*S. mutans*	*S. sobrinus*
Production of:		
β-glucosidase	+	–
α-galactosidase	+	–
Acid from:		
Arbutin	+	–
Inulin	+	d
Lactose	+	d
Mannitol	+	d
N-acetylglucosamine	+	–
Raffinose	+	–
Hydrolysis of:		
Aesculin	+	–
Arginine	–	–

Key:
+ = >90% of strains positive.
– = <10% of strains positive.
d = 50–90% of strains positive.
Source: Beighton *et al.* (1991b).
Reproduced with permission: Munksgaard International Publishers Ltd.

yet they may have different associations with dental caries due to different cariogenic properties (de Soet *et al.*, 1991).

The intra-oral distribution of the streptococci has been extensively studied (Frandsen *et al.*, 1991). Different species form different proportions of the flora on the different intra-oral sur-faces (Table 2.2). *S. salivarius* is isolated primarily from the tongue and saliva; *S. mutans* is isolated from the dental plaque, saliva and from the dorsum of the tongue; *S. oralis*, *S. sanguis* and *S. mitis*, which are associated with endocarditis and septicaemia in neutropaenic patients, may be isolated from all intra-oral surfaces (Bouvet *et al.*, 1994; Douglas *et al.*, 1993; Beighton *et al.*, 1994). Members of the 'milleri group', and *S. intermedius* in particular, are associated with liver and brain abscesses. The 'milleri group' are also isolated from oral abscesses and from urogenital infections; *S. anginosus* is more frequently isolated than *S. intermedius* and *S. constellatus* (Whiley *et al.*, 1990). The mechanisms underlying the intra-oral distributions of these species may be related to the presence of specific surface receptors on the surface of the bacteria and on the host surfaces to which they adhere (Gibbons, 1996).

2.2.2   Actinomyces and related genera

The Actinomyces and related genera form a significant proportion of the microflora of all intra-oral sites. These genera may be differentiated, in the laboratory, from other Gram-positive rods on the basis of significant physiological differences (Table 2.4). The identification of these bacteria to the genus level is not too difficult and is based on the production of fatty acids from glucose. However, their identification to the spe-

Table 2.4 Differentiation of Actinomyces and related genera

Genus	Aerobic growth	Catalase	Nitrate reduction	Acid end-products	Mol% G + C of the DNA
Actinomyces	d	d	d	ALS	58–68
Bifidobacterium	–	–	–	AL(S)	57–64
Corynebacterium	+	+	+	Alps	55–57
Eubacterium	–	–	d	(ALPBiBC)	30–40
Lactobacilli	d	–	–	Las	35–53
Propionibacterium	d	d	d	APLS	59–66
Rothia	+	+	+	ALs	65–69

Key:
+ = >90% positive.
− = <10% positive.
d = 11–89% positive.
A = acetic acid; L = lactic acid; S = succininc acid; P = propionic acid; B = butyric acid; iB = isobutryic acid; C = caproic acid.
Uppercase indicates major acid production and lowercase indicates minor acid production.
Acids in brackets may be produced by individual species within the genus. Some species of *Eubacterium* do not produce detectable levels of acids in broth.
Mol% G + C of the DNA is the mole percentage of the DNA composed of guaninine and cytosine.

cies level is time-consuming and not always possible in a routine microbiology laboratory.

The genus Actinomyces is the most numerous of the Gram-positive rods isolated from the human oral cavity and has undergone extensive taxonomic reorganisation in recent years (Johnson *et al.*, 1990). The human oral species are now recognised as *A. naeslundii* (containing genospecies 1, 2 and serotype WVA963), *A. georgiae*, *A. israelii*, *A. meyeri*, *A. gerencseriae* and *A. odontolyticus*; these species may be differentiated using a short set of biochemical reactions described by Johnson *et al.* (1990). Isolates identified as *A. naeslundii* cannot be identified to the genospecies level, except with DNA-DNA hybridisation or using genospecies specific antisera. The human strains of Actinomyces previously identified as *A. viscosus* on the basis of their ability to produce catalase are now included in the species *A. naeslundii*; the name *A. viscosus* is now confined to strains of animal origin.

Actinomyces spp. are isolated from the oral cavities of marsupials and mammals (omnivores and carnivores) and form part of the basic dental plaque flora. They are the most numerous genus in the oral cavity. *Actinomyces* spp. have been investigated in terms of their role in root caries in the elderly.

Propionibacterium spp. are present in dental plaque as a minor component of the dental plaque flora *P. propionica* (previously *Arachnia propionica*), *P. acnes*, *P. granulosum* and *P. avidum* are the major species isolated from the human oral cavity, sometimes in association with carious dentine.

Rothia dentocariosa is a single species genus and may be isolated as a component of newly formed dental plaque. *Corynebacterium (Bacterionema) matruchotii*, which is unusual in forming whip handle shaped cells, has a tendency to become mineralised and may be associated with calculus formation on the teeth.

Bifidobacterium spp. are not usually considered in studies of the dental plaque flora, due to the perceived difficulties in their isolation. However, they may be confused with *Actinomyces* spp., and their presence must be considered, especially in relation to the caries process because bifidobacteria are capable of growth at low pH.

2.2.3 Lactobacilli

The lactobacilli are capable of growing at low pH, they are aciduric, and are routinely isolated in the laboratory on media at pH 5. 2 (Rogosa Agar) supplemented with acetic acid. This medium is very selective and in most studies the lactobacilli are enumerated as a group with no attempt to identify the individual species. The main reasons for this are the great number of species (Schleifer and Ludwig, 1996; Dicks *et al.*, 1996) that may be encountered, and the absence of cheap and reliable schemes for their identification. The major oral species include *Acidophilus*, *Brevis*, *Casei subsp. casei*, *Fermentum*, *Gasseri*, *Oris*, *Parabuchneri*, *Zeae*, *Plantarum*, *Salivarius* subsp. *salivarius* and *Salivarius* subsp. *salicium*. In most instances, however, the numbers or proportions of this genus in saliva or dental plaque samples are regarded as indicators of poor oral hygiene, excessive intake of fermentable carbohydrate and/or increased caries risk. The role of individual species in the caries process has not been extensively studied.

2.2.4 Gram-negative cocci

The Gram-negative cocci in the oral cavity are mainly neisseria and veillonella. The neisseria are aerobic organisms isolated from all intra-oral surfaces and are identified as oxidase and catalase positive cocci. They may be identified to the species level using tests for acid production from a range of carbohydrates.

The veillonella are anaerobic cocci, unable to produce acid from carbohydrates. They are identified on the basis of their ability to utilise lactate for the production of energy with the formation of acetate and propionate as end-products. Veillonella may proliferate in dental plaque containing high numbers of streptococci which produce lactic acid from carbohydrates. The lactic acid produced is used in the growth of veillonella, and this may consequently reduce the extent of enamel demineralisation (van der Hoeven *et al.*, 1978; Noorda *et al.*, 1988).

2.2.5 Aerobic and Capnophilic Gram-negative rods

These include the genera Haemophilus, Eikonella, Actinobacillus and Capnocytophaga. Of these genera, it is *Actinobacillus actinomycetemcomitans* which may be most associated with human oral diseases: juvenile periodontitis and adult chronic periodontitis. These organisms are routinely isolated in the laboratory using a selective culture medium (Slots, 1982).

2.2.6 Anaerobic Gram-negative bacteria

This groups of organisms is complicated and encompasses primarily members of the genera Prevotella, Porphyromonas, Campylobacter, Fusobacterium, Wolinella and Treponema (Vandamme *et al.*, 1991; Paster *et al.*, 1994; Table 2.5). They require anaerobic conditions for their isolation and growth in the laboratory, they are oxygen sensitive, and are isolated mainly from the periodontal pockets around the teeth. They may be associated with periodontal diseases (Slots and Genco, 1984; Slots and Listgarten, 1988; Tanner, 1991), dental abscesses (Lewis *et al.*, 1988) and root canal infections (Sundqvist, 1992). However, they are all members of the normal oral flora and cannot be considered to be infectious agents in the strict sense.

It is the capnophilic and anaerobic bacteria present in the periodontal pocket that are most associated with the presence of active periodontal disease, which may be indicated by the presence of spontaneous gingival bleeding upon probing with a periodontal probe or, perhaps more correctly, the active resorption of the bone supporting the affected tooth. The specific bacterial species mediating the destruction of the periodontal bone is unclear, as periodontal diseases are associated with mixed anaerobic infections in which the proportions of individual species vary. The microflora of periodontal sites showing active destructive progression has been investigated extensively (Moore *et al.*, 1991).

The major nutrient sources for the microflora in the periodontal sulcus are the host tissue components, including serum glycoproteins and proteins that enter the sulcus through the epithelial cell surface of the sulcus. There is no evidence that the components of the diet directly influence the microflora of the periodontal sulcus, although localised microbial expansion may occur in association with the impaction of foods into the sulcus resulting in gingival swelling and bleeding.

2.2.7 Yeasts

The yeast most frequently isolated from the oral cavity is *Candida albicans* and it may be identified in the laboratory by its ability to form germ tubes and produce N-acetylhexosaminidase activity (Perry and Miller, 1987). The range of other species isolated from the oral cavity may include *C. tropicalis*, *C. (Torulopsis) glabrata*, *C. parapsilosis*, *C. krusei*, *C. magnoliae*, *C. lusitaniae*, *C. famata*, *C. kefir* and *Sacchromyces cerevisiae* (Budtz-Jorgensen *et al.*, 1975; Beighton *et al.*, 1995). In the laboratory, yeasts are grown routinely on Sabouraud Dextrose Agar, but new media have been developed that permit the presumptive identification of several yeast species on primary isolation. Confirmation was gained by the use of commercial testing kits (Odds *et al.*, 1994). Saliva samples are examined for yeasts in relation to dental caries and to determine the frequency and amount of consumption of fermentable sugars by individual patients. Candida are also associated with denture sore mouth and angular chelitis, and oral infections due to *C. albicans* are common in patients with AIDS.

2.3 THE ACQUISITION OF BACTERIA

The oral cavity prior to birth is sterile until passage down the birth canal where microorganisms with the potential to colonise its mucosal surfaces are encountered. The oral flora of the newborn child is composed primarily of streptococci. *S. oralis*, *S. mitis* and *S. salivarius* form the majority of the streptococcal flora (Pearce *et al.*,

Table 2.5 Differential characteristics of the major genera of Gram-negative anaerobic rods isolated from the human oral cavity

Genus	Species	Genus characteristics
Prevotella	*intermedia* *nigrescens* *bivia* *buccae* *buccalis* *corporis* *denticola* *dentalis* *disiens* *loeschii* *melaninogenicus* *oralis* *oris*	Pleomorphic rods with blunt ends, saccharolytic producing mainly acetic and succinic acids and occasionally lesser amounts of isobutyric, isovaleric and lactic acids from glucose. May be pigmented.
Porphyromon	*gingivalis* *endodontalis* *levii*	Pleomorphic rods with blunt ends, asaccharolytic producing mainly acetic, butyric and phenylacetic acids and occasionally isobutyric, isovaleric, propionic and succinic acids from peptides. Pigmented.
Fusobacterium	*nucleatum* *alocis* *periodonticum*	Regular, blunt ended cells, assaccharolytic producing mainly butyric and isolvaleric acids from peptides.
Selenomonas	*noxia* *flueggei* *artemidis* *infelix* *sputigena*	Curved to helical rods, motile with active tumbling, saccharolyic producing mainly acetic and propionic acids.
Wolinella	*succinogens*	Mainly helical cells, motile and require succinate for growth.
Campylobacter	*rectus* *curvus* *gracilis* *showae*	Slender, spirally curved motile rods microaerophilic, carbohydrates not fermented.
Treponema	*denticola* *pectinovorum* *vincentii* *scoliodentium* *macrodentium*	Motile

1995). Recently, Könönen *et al.* (1992) determined the occurrence of Gram-negative anaerobes in 30 infants prior to tooth eruption (mean age 3 months, range 1–7 months). *Prevotella melaninogenica* was the most frequently isolated anaerobe, found in 70% of the infants. The other common anaerobes were *Fusobacterium nucleatum*, *Veillonella* spp., '*Bacteroides gracilis*' and non-pigmented *Prevotella* spp., found in 60, 57, 23 and 57% of the infants, respectively. *Leptotrichia* spp., microaerophilic *Capnocytophaga* spp., *Prevotella loescheii* and *Prevotella intermedia* were found in 17, 13 and 7% of the infants, respectively, while *Actinobacillus actinomycetemcomitans* was not detected. These data clearly indicate that various anaerobic bacterial species readily colonise the mouth of infants prior to tooth eruption.

The most significant change that takes place in the acquisition of bacteria in the oral cavity is the eruption of the teeth. The teeth represent new surfaces to colonise and it is only upon the eruption of teeth that the mutans streptococci (*S. mutans* and *S. sobrinus*) are isolated from the oral cavity (Grindefjord *et al.*, 1995b). These bacteria are not usually found in the mouth until after the eruption of the lateral incisor teeth (Berkowitz *et al.*, 1975). In exceptional cases usually associated with excessive consumption of fermentable carbohydrates, they may be acquired very soon after the eruption of the first teeth (central incisors). DNA fingerprinting techniques, bacteriocin typing and serotyping, all show that mutans first colonising infants are acquired from the child's mother or main carer (Li and Caufield, 1995). In extensive longitudinal studies in Scandinavia, it has been shown that the earlier the mutans streptococci are acquired by the child, the greater the likelihood that the child will develop tooth decay (Kolher *et al.*,

1984; Kohler and Andreen, 1994). The adult flora remains relatively constant. Changes occur in old age when changes in the host immune system, reduced salivary flow rate and wearing of dentures, may facilitate the colonisation of the mouth by enteric bacteria and increased populations of yeasts, mutans streptococci and lactobacilli (Beighton *et al.*, 1991; Marsh *et al.*, 1992; Terpenning *et al.*, 1993).

2.4 GROWTH OF DENTAL PLAQUE BACTERIA

The nutrients available for the growth of bacteria on the teeth derive from the components of the diet, saliva and gingival crevicular fluid and shed epithelial cells. For the majority of the time, the intervals between meals and snacks, the principal nutrient source available to the dental plaque bacteria on the exposed surfaces of the teeth are the glycoproteins (mucins) of the salivary secretions. For the bacteria in the gingival crevice, the major sources of nutrients are the tissue exudates containing serum glycoproteins and proteins, and the epithelial cells of the gingival surface; dietary components do not usually enter the gingival crevice. Dental plaque bacteria produce enzymes: (a) glycosidase; neuraminidase (sialidase), α-fucosidase, α-mannosidase, β-mannosidase, β-N-acetylglucosaminidase, β-N-acetylgalactosaminidase and β-galactosidase which remove sugars from the side-chains; and (b) proteases (amino-, diamino- and endo-peptidases) which degrade the protein core of mucins (MG1 and MG2) (Levine *et al.*, 1987). They also degrade glycosylated proline-rich proteins (PRPs) (Oho *et al.*, 1992) in saliva and serum glycoproteins found in the gingival crevice. These enzymes are produced by dental plaque bacteria all the time, but the levels are increased when food, which usually includes many essential aminoacids and peptides, is unavailable (Beighton *et al.*, 1986; Smith and Beighton, 1986). The bacteria synergistically degrade salivary mucins and serum glycoproteins; different bacteria exhibit different enzyme activities and different growth requirements (Carlsson *et al.*, 1984; Sundqvist *et al.*, 1985; van der Hoeven *et al.*, 1990; ter Steeg *et al.*, 1987; Bradshaw *et al.*, 1994). Furthermore, the growth rates (doubling times of 2–4 hours) of dental plaque bacteria in fasted and fed laboratory animals are not different, indicating that salivary mucins provide sufficient nutrients for bacterial growth (Beckers and van der Hoeven, 1984; Beighton and Hayday, 1986).

The clinical significance of these observations is apparent in leukaemic children who, following bone marrow transplantation, are so unwell that they eat very little and this has the effect of selecting for an oral flora which is composed predominantly of those bacteria best able to utilise salivary mucins for growth. The levels of *S. oralis* and *S. mitis* increase from 5% to almost 50% of the flora within 5 days of the bone marrow transplant (Lucas *et al.*, 1997). The composition of the carbohydrate side-chains on salivary mucins and serum glycoproteins are very similar, so that the entry of the bacteria proliferating in the oral cavity into the circulation may result in their growth in the bloodstream. *S. oralis* and *S. mitis* are among the major causes of septicaemia, endocarditis and acute respiratory infections (Beighton *et al.*, 1994; Bochud *et al.*, 1994).

The addition of sugar (sucrose) to the diet does not increase the rate of growth of bacteria in dental plaque. However, the bacteria in the plaque will produce extra-cellular polysaccharides (glucans and fructans) which will effectively bulk up the plaque, increasing the mass of plaque on the dentition (Staat *et al.*, 1975).

3

FOOD COMPONENTS RELEVANT TO ORAL HEALTH

General good health depends on a proper balance of all nutrients and, in this sense, an overview of all food components may be considered relevant to oral health. However, deficiencies and excesses of some nutrients have specific manifestations in the oral hard or soft tissues. This chapter is a brief overview of nutrients in food with a special emphasis on those thought to be particularly related to the development and maintenance of oral tissues. These include components with systemic or local effects on hard tissues: energy, carbohydrates, protein, vitamin D, calcium, phosphorus, magnesium, fluoride and the trace elements selenium, strontium, lithium and molybdenum. Those implicated in systemic or local effects on the soft tissues include the vitamins A, C, E and other antioxidant nutrients, as well as folate and other B vitamins, the minerals iron and zinc and alcohol.

Plant and animal foods contain nutrients, other biologically active substances, inert substances, and some natural toxicants and pollutants. The main components of diet are the macronutrients, carbohydrate, fat and protein. These form the bulk of the foods, apart from water, and provide all the energy which is their common denominator. Vitamins and minerals (micronutrients) are present in very small quantities and are equally essential for specific physiological functions. Essential nutrients are those that must be supplied from the diet as they cannot be formed from other substances in the body. Non-essential nutrients are those that exist in foods but can also be made in the body. Vitamin C is an example that is essential for humans but non-essential for most other animals, who can make it from glucose.

3.1 WATER

Water is the largest component of most foodstuffs, both plant and animal. The human body is about 70% water, as is meat. The water content of plant foods ranges from 5% in nuts and oilseeds, 10% in grains and pulses, to 80% in potatoes and 95% in watermelons.

3.2 ENERGY

Energy is needed for activity, but most of the energy consumed from food is used for basal metabolism, the chemical processes that keep the heart beating, the blood circulating and the brain functioning. Energy is measured in kilocalories or kilojoules (1 kcal = 4.18 kJ) and adults require approximately 1500–3000 kcals per day depending on gender, body size and activity level. This is obtained from the major components of food: carbohydrates, fat, protein and alcohol. Vitamins and minerals provide no energy. Pure carbohydrate provides approximately 4 kcal/g, fat 9 kcal/g, protein 4 kcal/g (and alcohol 7 kcal/g).

3.3 CARBOHYDRATES

Carbohydrates supply most of the energy intake of the majority of the world's population. These are derived almost exclusively from plant foods, as the carbohydrate content of most foods of animal origin is negligible, except for lactose (milk sugar). In the report by the UK Committee on the Medical Aspects of Food Policy (COMA) on Dietary Sugars and Human Disease (DH, 1989), a new classification of sugars was introduced, based on their location in foods: intrinsic sugars were defined as those within plant cells, such as in whole fruit, whereas, extrinsic sugars were those free in solutions such as fruit juices and honey, or added during food preparation (recipe sugars) or at the time of consumption (table sugars). To distinguish lactose from other sugars in solution the term non-milk extrinsic sugars (NMES) was devised. The purpose of this classification was to separate those sugars considered to be important as a cause of dental decay (NMES) from those that were negligible causes (lactose and intrinsic sugars). The Committee recommended that total non-milk extrinsic sugars in the average diet should be limited to 11% of food energy (or 10% of total energy intake, which assumes some energy intake from alcohol).

This classification has since engendered considerable debate based on the lack of methods of chemical analysis to distinguish between them, and on the lack of difference in physiological effects (Johnson *et al*. 1996; Rugg-Gunn and Cottrell, 1997). This debate has highlighted the difficulty of making a clear distinction between intrinsic and extrinsic sugars, as intrinsic sugars become extrinsic to a variable extent when plant cell walls are disrupted during food preparation and cooking, or when chewed. One example would be dried fruit such as figs, which contain 53% sugars, mainly glucose (29%) and fructose (23%); these sugars are originally intrinsic, but become extrinsic and more concentrated on drying. Lactose was singled out by COMA as a special case of extrinsic sugar, as it was considered to be of low importance in dental decay, and is limited to dairy foods in which calcium provides caries protection. The FAO/WHO Expert Consultation on Carbohydrate held in April 1997 (FAO/WHO, 1997) agreed to classify carbohydrates only on the basis of chemical structure (monosaccharides, disaccharides and sugar alcohols, oligosaccharides and polysaccharides), as extrinsic and intrinsic sugars cannot be distinguished in practice, and this distinction is made only in the UK. Other commonly used descriptors of the source of sugars in foods are 'natural' and 'added' which also cannot be distinguished after the food is prepared.

Nevertheless, although the terminology is debated, the basic concept is valid, and sugars that are free or added to the diet have a critical role in causing dental caries. Currently, most added sugar is sucrose which therefore forms the bulk of sugars in the diet, but other sugars, such as glucose, fructose, invert sugars and maltodextrins, are increasingly used in manufactured food products. It is not known to what extent these other sugars would be related to dental decay if they were consumed in similar quantities to sucrose, but they are likely to be equivalent.

Carbohydrates are classified according to the complexity of single sugar units (monosaccharides) that are linked together. Both mono- and disaccharides are sweet, but glucose is only half as sweet as sucrose. The chemical structure of some sugars is shown in Figure 3.1.

3.3.1 Monosaccharides

Monosaccharides normally contain three to seven carbon atoms with hydrogen and oxygen attached, and are named trioses, tetroses, pentoses, hexoses and heptoses, respectively. The hexoses are the most important in the diet, and can exist either as straight chains or in a ring structure. Hexoses include glucose, which is not abundant in free form in natural foods, but is found in small amounts in fruits and vegetables. It is one of the main constituents of honey and can be manufactured by the hydrolysis of starch. Fructose is found in fruits, vegetables and honey. Galactose is found in milk as a component of the disaccharide lactose.

3.3.2 Disaccharides

Combinations of two simple sugars are the disaccharides. Sucrose is the most commonly consumed sugar, and is extracted from either sugar beet or cane. Table sugar is 99.9% pure sucrose and when incorporated in recipes is the main source of sucrose in the diet. Sucrose is also present in fruit and vegetables. It is broken down into glucose and fructose as it is digested in the intestine. Lactose is formed from glucose and galactose and is only found in milk. Maltose consisting of two molecules of glucose is present in sprouted (malted) wheat and barley, from which malt extract is produced for brewing and for malted food products. Trehalose, or mushroom sugar, is another disaccharide composed of two molecules of glucose and constitutes up to 15% of the dry matter of mushrooms.

3.3.3 Oligosaccharides

Short chains of monosaccharide sugars are called oligosaccharides. These include the manufactured maltodextrins and glucose syrups as well as raffinose, stachyose and verbascose, which are found mainly in legumes such as peas and beans and fructans found in cereals, onions, garlic, asparagus and Jerusalem artichokes, which also contain the longer chain fructan, inulin. The latter are not broken down by human digestive enzymes and so pass into the large intestine, where they are fermented by bacteria, producing short-chain fatty acids and gases leading to flatulence.

3.3.4 Sugar alcohols

Sugar alcohol is the chemical name of specific forms of sugars found in nature and prepared commercially—not to be confused with the alco-

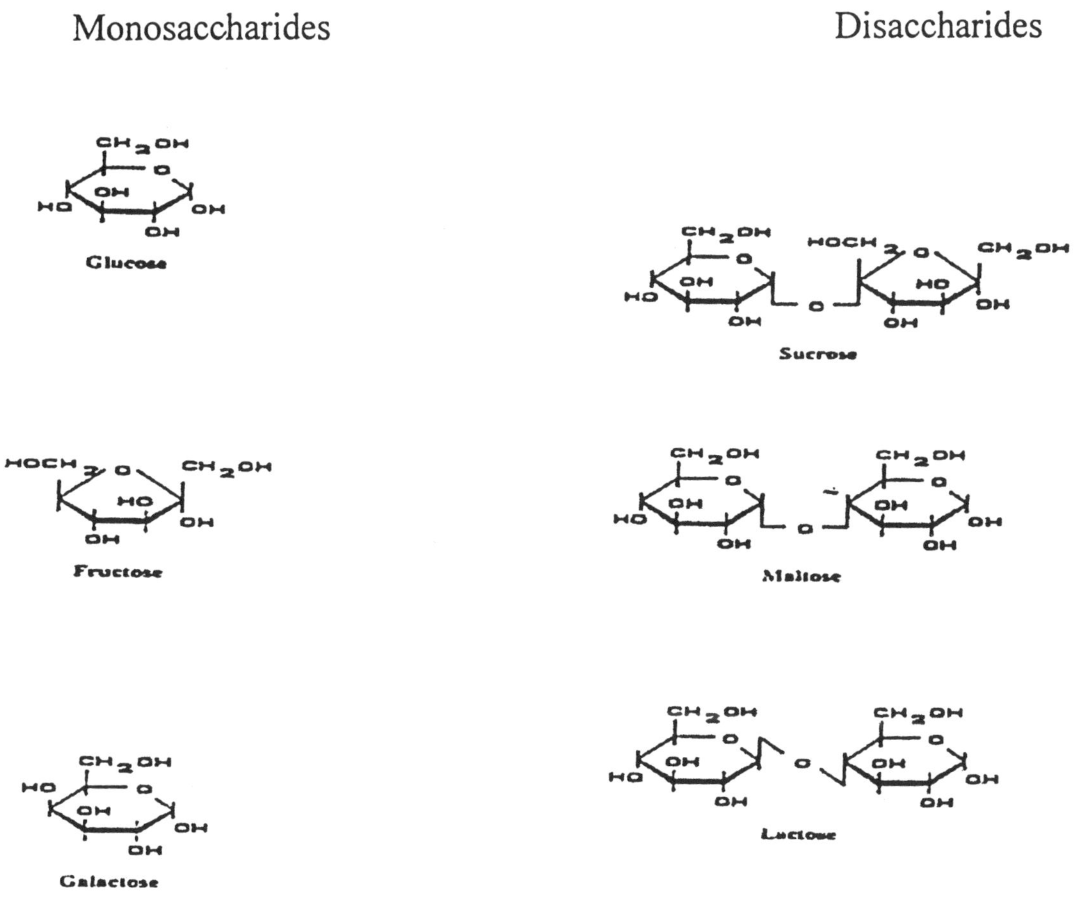

Monosaccharides

Glucose

Fructose

Galactose

Disaccharides

Sucrose

Maltose

Lactose

Figure 3.1   The chemical structure of some sugars.
Source: Bender (1993). Reprinted with permission of Taylor and Francis Ltd.

hol ethanol, prepared by the fermentation of various carbohydrates. Sugar alcohols include xylitol found in birch, sorbitol found in fruits such as cherries, mannitol, extracted from a seaweed, and inositol present in many foods, particularly cereal bran. Sorbitol and xylitol are produced commercially for use as sweeteners in foods and drinks for diabetics, because they are absorbed from the intestine more slowly and so have less effect on blood glucose levels than sucrose. They are less sweet than sucrose and have a cool mouth feel. They are also used in 'tooth friendly' sweets and chewing gums because the bacteria in the mouth cannot use sugar alcohols to produce the acid which causes tooth decay. Inositol combines with phosphate to form phytic acid, present in many plant foods, which is important nutritionally as it impairs the absorption of calcium and iron in the intestine.

3.3.5   Polysaccharides

The polysaccharides are long chains of monosaccharides, but are not sweet. Starch is the major polysaccharide and form of carbohydrate in the human diet, and the main storage form of energy in cereals, root crops and plantains. It consists of two types of chains of glucose molecules: amylose is an unbranched chain; amylopectin is highly branched. Starch granules from different plants contain varying proportions of amylose and amylopectin. Starch is insoluble in water and therefore not easily digested until cooked, causing it to swell. Recooling reduces digestibility, forming 'resistant starch'. Other polysaccharides include cellulose and gums.

3.3.6   Dietary fibre

Dietary fibre is a term that has been used loosely to describe the plant material that is resistant to digestion in the human intestine. This could include lignin, a woody substance that is not a carbohydrate, some forms of starch and other components. However, to characterise it chemically, and allow a better understanding of the effects of various components on digestion and metabolism, it is now generally accepted to define it as non-starch polysaccharide (NSP).

NSP includes cellulose (insoluble) which is the main component of plant cell walls, and non-cellulose polysaccharides (mainly water soluble), including: pectin, which is extracted commercially and used as a gelling agent in jams; β-glucans, of which cereals such as oats and barley are a good source, and which may explain the cholesterol lowering effect of oat bran; gums such as guar gum and gum arabic, which are extracted commercially and used in the food industry as emulsifiers, stabilisers and thickeners; mucilages such as alginates, carrageen and agar which are found in seaweeds and other algae, and used as a thickener in dairy products and confectionery.

Whole grain cereals are especially rich sources of NSP, mainly insoluble in wheat, maize and rice, whereas, a significant proportion is soluble in oats, barley and rye. In vegetables the soluble and insoluble fractions are approximately equal, but in fruits the proportions are widely variable. Dietary fibre, especially insoluble fibre such as wheat bran, decreases intestinal transit time and increases fecal bulk. Soluble NSP (pectins, gums, etc.) can be effective in reducing cholesterol levels in the blood. Low intake of dietary fibre, common in industrialised societies, is a factor in several diseases such as constipation, colorectal cancer, coronary heart disease and gallstones.

3.4 FAT

In the UK diet, and that of other industrialised countries, approximately 40% of the energy comes from fats and oils, but intakes can be as low as 10% in some non-industrialised countries. Dietary fats and oils are chemically mainly triglycerides, molecules composed of three fatty acids attached to a glycerol core. Triglycerides are an important form of energy storage in both animals and plants. Fatty acids are classified as saturated, monounsaturated or polyunsaturated, referring to the extent to which hydrogen fills the available carbon bonds. Saturated fatty acids have all bonds filled, monounsaturates have one bond unfilled, and polyunsaturated fatty acids have several unfilled. These groups have different properties and functions; the longer the chain length and the more saturated, the harder the fat. Unsaturated fats react more readily with oxygen and become rancid. Saturated fats are more stable for storage.

In general, fats from animal sources contain mainly saturated (40–60%) and monounsaturated fatty acids (30–50%), with few polyunsaturated (<10%), while plant foods contain fats that are mainly polyunsaturated (40–60%) and monounsaturated (30–40%) with smaller proportions of saturated fatty acids. There are a few exceptions such as coconut oil and palm oil which are highly saturated (90 and 50%), while poultry and game have more polyunsaturated fatty acids, especially turkey (35%). Milk fat contains a high proportion of short-chain saturated fatty acids.

3.5 PROTEIN

Protein constitutes 10–15% of the energy in almost all human diets. It is important in the structure of all cells in the body, as well as enzymes, molecules that transport substances in the blood and some hormones. There is a large variety of proteins in both food and the body with different composition and function. All proteins are composed of about 20 different amino acids which are molecules that have the common features of containing nitrogen (about 16%), carbon, oxygen and hydrogen. The body is able to synthesise some amino acids in the liver (non-essential amino acids), but others have to be obtained from food (essential amino acids). Amino acids can be linked together to form peptides ranging from dipeptides with two amino acids, to polypeptides with up to thousands. Proteins are made up of polypeptide chains, folded into structures with different shapes depending on their function.

Protein deficiency is unlikely to occur except when total food intake is too low, or where the diet, especially a weaning diet, consists almost entirely of plant food with a particularly low protein content in relation to total calories, such as cassava or plantain. Protein energy malnutrition (PEM) is the term used to describe the effects of diets inadequate in total quantity rather than in relation to deficiencies of specific nutrients. Delayed eruption of the teeth has been associated with PEM in childhood.

3.6 ALCOHOL

Alcohol is not a component of any natural plant or animal food, however, in almost all cultures it is produced from whichever plants are grown in abundance, and it can provide a considerable source of energy in the diet. In some cultures, milk is fermented to an alcoholic drink. Alcohol is produced by yeast fermentation of carbohydrates from a wide variety of sources: beer from barley; vodka from potato; rum from sugar; palm wine from the sweet sap of palm trees; whisky from barley; and wine from grapes. Excessive long-term alcohol consumption can lead to malnutrition by displacing other foods and their specific nutrients from the diet, and by damaging gastrointestinal and liver function. In chronic liver disease deficiencies occur in the fat soluble vitamins, some water soluble vitamins, especially thiamin and folate, and some minerals especially iron. High alcohol consumption is a risk factor for oral cancer and acts synergistically with cigarette smoking (see Chapter 10). The carcinogenic potential may be related to the local irritant effect on the oral mucosa, and also to a low consumption of fruits and vegetables associated with high alcohol intakes, and a loss of their cancer protective effect. The average intake of energy from alcohol in the UK is 6.9% for men and 2.8% for women (Gregory et al., 1990), but heavy drinkers can derive up to half or more of their energy from alcohol.

3.7 MICRONUTRIENTS

Vitamins are substances required in very small amounts, μg or mg per day, to maintain normal metabolism. The body is unable to synthesise them and so they must be obtained from food. By definition, vitamins are essential nutrients. However, two are essential only under specific conditions as they can be synthesised to a certain extent in the body: vitamin D and niacin. Vitamin D is formed in skin exposed to sunlight, and is essential in the diet only if exposure to sunlight is inadequate. Therefore, it is considered by some to be a hormone rather than a vitamin. Niacin can be formed from the essential amino acid tryptophan, and it is now thought that the amount formed is as important as the preformed niacin obtained from the diet. Vitamins can have adverse effects at high doses, especially the fat-soluble vitamins that can accumulate in the liver and fat tissues. However, when consumed in plant foods there is no risk of excess, and the problem only arises from the over use of vitamin supplements, or from high intakes of liver from animals in which vitamin A has accumulated from their food.

All nutritionally important minerals have to be provided in the diet as elements cannot be converted in the body, and many are known to be essential for specific functions. Those required in larger amounts (g/day) are calcium, magnesium and phosphorus which form the structure of bones and teeth, as well as having other metabolic functions, and sodium, chloride and potassium which are important for the mainten-

ance of the normal composition of fluids outside and inside the cells of the body. Others required in smaller amounts (mg or μg/day) are associated with specific enzymes or hormones, such as copper, iron, molybdenum, selenium, zinc, chromium, cobalt, iodine, magnesium and manganese. Others are known to be essential but their function is not yet known: silicon, vanadium, nickel and tin. Some have beneficial effects but are not established as essential such as fluoride and lithium.

The function of vitamins and minerals of particular relevance to oral health are discussed briefly in this section. Some vitamins and minerals are present in many foods in available form, such as vitamin E and pantothenic acid and so deficiencies are rare, others are concentrated in certain foods, such as vitamins A and C, or often occur in less available forms, such as iron, and so deficiencies are more frequent.

3.7.1 Fat soluble vitamins

Vitamins are classified into fat soluble (A, D, E and K) or water soluble (B and C vitamins). Deficiencies of the fat soluble vitamins can occur if the level of fat in the diet is so low that absorption is impaired. Conversely adverse effects of high intakes may occur mainly with this group as they can be stored and accumulate in the body.

3.7.1.1 Vitamin A

The term vitamin A covers two groups of compounds: retinol or pre-formed vitamin A, which is found only in animal foods; and the carotenes, from which retinol can be formed in the body, which are found in green, yellow and orange coloured fruits and vegetables. Carotenes are converted to retinol with varying efficiency. Beta-carotene has the highest vitamin A activity: 6 μg is equivalent to 1 μg retinol. For others such as α-carotene and cryptoxanthine, 12 μg is equivalent to 1 μg retinol. Retinol is stored in the liver of animals and excess liver consumption can lead to toxicity. However, this risk does not exist with the precursor carotenes, as their conversion to retinol is regulated.

Vitamin A deficiency is one of the most widespread micronutrient deficiencies worldwide, but only in less developed countries. The well known function of vitamin A is the metabolism of the visual pigments of the eye. Deficiency of vitamin A leads first to night blindness and subsequently to complete blindness. Another extremely important function is in the control of cell differentiation so that deficiency leads to abnormalities of the skin and mucosa, and poorer resistance to respiratory and gastrointestinal disease.

Carotenoids have a separate function as antioxidants and are now thought to be important in resistance to cell damage by the many substances that produce 'free radicals'. These are highly reactive molecules that result in the oxidative damage associated with ageing, heart disease and cancer.

3.7.1.2 *Vitamin D*

Vitamin D (calciferol) is essential for the proper formation of the skeleton and for the regulation of mineral metabolism. Exposure to ultraviolet light, either from sunlight or artificial sources, produces vitamin D_3 (cholecalciferol) from 7-dehydrocholesterol in the skin. The other major form is vitamin D_2 (ergocalciferol) produced by UV light on ergosterol in plants, which is present in small amounts from natural sources but is the major synthetic form used in human and animal foods. Cholecalciferol is widely distributed in animals, and amounts are dependent on the vitamin D content of their diet and exposure to sunlight. Fish liver and fish liver oils are rich sources of vitamin D, but most foods only contain low amounts, and some countries require fortification of food such as milk or margarine with either form of the vitamin. Absorption is decreased by the phytate content of plant foods. Human requirements can be met if the skin is exposed to sufficient sunlight, but the effectiveness of vitamin D production depends on the area of the skin and the time exposed, the season, latitude, skin colour and age. The capacity of the skin to synthesise vitamin D_3 is reduced in elderly people, and so vitamin D is considered an essential dietary nutrient in this group.

The vitamin is metabolised into active forms whose main physiological role is to maintain calcium and phosphorus homeostasis by stimulating their absorption from the intestine and reabsorption in the kidney and controlling the mineralisation and demineralisation of bone and dental hard tissues. Deficiencies can lead to rickets in children and osteomalacia in adults. Deficiencies occur in communities where people, especially women and children, do not go out in the sun, and the diet consists largely of unrefined cereals and contains few animal products. In the UK, rickets was common at the beginning of the twentieth century in industrial cities such as Glasgow, but has been virtually eliminated except for a few cases in Asian communities where the requisite conditions exist. Excessive

intakes, to which young children are the most susceptible, lead to the deposition of calcium in soft tissues and subsequent cardiovascular and kidney damage.

3.7.1.3 *Vitamin E*

Vitamin E is a highly effective antioxidant, and has an important role in protecting polyunsaturated fatty acids and other components of cell membranes from oxidation by free radicals. It may have other functions such as anti-inflammatory properties and the stimulation of the immune response. Vegetable oils are major sources of vitamin E in the diet. The quantities required to prevent overt deficiency with signs of damage to cell membranes are less than the intake needed to reduce the risk of cancers, coronary heart disease and other degenerative diseases.

3.7.2 Water soluble vitamins

On a worldwide basis, deficiencies of B vitamins that were once common, such as pellagra (niacin deficiency) and beriberi (thiamin deficiency), have been almost eliminated through improved diets, better food processing and fortification, although during the 1980s they have reappeared in the expanding population of refugees in the world, due to the use of emergency food supplies unsuitable for long term feeding. The B vitamins which remain problematic are vitamin B_2 (riboflavin) in communities that do not consume rich sources such as milk, and folate and vitamin B_{12}.

3.7.2.1 *Riboflavin*

Riboflavin deficiency rarely occurs alone, and usually with other vitamin deficiencies. Many of the oral and genital lesions originally included in the signs of pellagra, were found to be due to riboflavin deficiency: angular cheilitis, glossitis, lip fissures, and seborrhoeic dermatitis in nasolabial folds and eyelids. It functions as a component of coenzymes that catalyse many oxidation-reduction reactions, including the conversion of tryptophan to niacin. Food sources are mainly animal, especially dairy and meat products. Grains naturally contain low levels, but fortified cereal and bakery products supply large amounts. In the UK milk and milk products provide 27% of riboflavin in the diet; meat and meat products 21%; cereal products 22% (mainly from breakfast cereals). Beverages provide 13% for men and 8% for women, the higher value for men being mainly from the contribution of beer (Gregory *et al.*, 1990).

3.7.2.2 *Folate and vitamin B_{12}*

Folate and vitamin B_{12} deficiencies both result in megaloblastic anaemia. This anaemia is characterised by large immature blood cells in contrast to the more common iron deficiency anaemia, where the blood cells are smaller than normal. Folate is the generic term for compounds that have nutritional properties and chemical structures similar to folic acid (pteroylglutamic acid). Folates act as coenzymes in amino acid metabolism and nucleic acid synthesis, so that a deficiency leads to impaired cell division and protein synthesis, consequently the effects are most noticeable in rapidly growing tissues. They are widely distributed in foods, with liver, yeast, leafy green vegetables, legumes and some fruits being especially rich sources. However, much may be destroyed in food processing and preparation. Deficiency of folate is not uncommon, especially in developing countries, despite its presence in most fresh foods, as it is easily oxidised. Pregnancy increases requirements, and if the mother's stores are low, neural tube defects such as spina bifida, can occur in the infant.

Vitamin B_{12} deficiency impairs normal cell division, and at a later stage demyelination of nerves occurs, resulting in anaemia, peripheral neuropathy, memory loss and dementia. As vitamin B_{12} is naturally present only in animal foods, this vitamin can be problematic amongst vegans, unless fortified foods or supplements are taken. Some fermented foods such as yeast products may provide small amounts of vitamin B_{12}, as microorganisms also form B_{12}. However, most vitamin B_{12} deficiency is not due to low levels in the diet, but to a pathological condition which reduces its absorption in the intestine. The metabolism of folate requires vitamin B_{12} and so the two vitamins are closely linked. Vitamin B_{12} deficiency results in secondary folate deficiency. Supplementation with folate would treat the resultant megaloblastic anaemia, but would mask the other effects of vitamin B_{12} deficiency including degeneration of the spinal cord. It is therefore important to eliminate vitamin B_{12} deficiency as a cause of megaloblastic anaemia before treating with additional folate.

3.7.2.3 *Niacin*

Pellagra, caused by niacin deficiency, was first recognised to occur in poor people on a corn (maize) based diet devoid of animal proteins. Maize contains very little niacin, in a form not readily available, and meat provides the amino acid tryptophan which can be converted to niacin. Pellagra also occurs with poor sorghum based diets. The disease was prevalent in Europe and southern USA after the introduction of maize, and is classically characterised by the three Ds: dermatitis, diarrhoea and dementia. The tongue is inflamed and a red rash occurs in areas of the skin exposed to the sun. Pellagra does not exist where maize is prepared in the traditional way by soaking in lime, which increases the bioavailability of niacin. Pellagra still occurs in parts of India and Africa associated with the consumption of sorghum based diets, and is also occasionally found in alcoholics.

3.7.2.4 *Vitamin C*

Vitamin C deficiency was a common problem in the past at the end of winter after months without fresh fruit and vegetables, but modern transport and storage systems have made fresh produce available the year round, and so signs of deficiency are uncommon. Deficiency can occur in groups such as the elderly or alcoholics, where intakes are low, and in infants fed exclusively on cow's milk.

The best defined role of vitamin C is in the hydroxylation of the amino acids proline and lysine in the formation of collagen in connective tissues, but it is also involved in a large number of reactions that affect the function of diverse systems such as neurotransmitters, immune responses, and wound healing. Vitamin C is an antioxidant and plays a role in the prevention of diseases such as coronary heart disease and certain cancers. Being a water soluble vitamin, it is excreted once the body tissues are saturated at intakes of about 100 mg/day and, therefore, there is no good evidence for the very high doses claimed to be beneficial in the treatment or prevention of cancer, or the common cold. Vitamin C is important in aiding the absorption of non-haem iron from the diet. In the UK, vegetables provide 46% of the vitamin C in the diet with potatoes the most important providing 16%; beverages provide 22%, mainly from fruit juice; and fruit and nuts provide 17%. Supplements provide on average 8 mg of vitamin C daily (11%) for men, and 11 mg (15%) for women (Gregory *et al.*, 1990).

3.7.3 **Minerals**

The minerals that have been associated with systemic or local effects on the oral hard or soft tissues are calcium, phosphorus, fluoride, iron, zinc, magnesium and the trace elements selenium, strontium, lithium and molybdenum. In general, inadequate mineral intakes occur where there is a particular deficiency in the soil, and the population consumes only locally grown products. In practice this is now rare, except for iodine deficiency, due to extensive commerce and mixed diets. Some minerals are lost in the milling of cereals and several countries require the fortification of flour with minerals, such as the UK, where calcium and iron are added to all wheat flours except wholemeal. Foods such as breakfast cereals are frequently fortified with iron and other minerals. Water is a variable source of minerals. The main mineral deficiencies are caused by excessive losses and poor absorption. Iron, iodine, calcium and zinc are the most problematic worldwide. Many minerals cause adverse effects in excess, but this is unlikely to occur with food, except where crops are grown on soil with very high selenium levels. Problems can also arise with inappropriate supplements or contamination of food or water. High intakes of fluoride can result in dental fluorosis, and very high intakes, where the fluoride content of the water supply is much greater than 1 ppm, may result in bone defects.

3.7.3.1 *Calcium*

The adult body contains approximately 1200 g calcium, of which 99% is in the skeleton. The remainder is in the extracellular fluids and cell membranes, where it has an essential role in nerve conduction, muscle contraction, blood clotting and membrane permeability, and is maintained within very narrow limits by several hormones.

Calcium requirements are especially high during rapid growth in infancy, adolescence and pregnancy, and during lactation. In many countries the main sources of calcium are milk and dairy products but in other countries milk is not consumed after childhood, and so calcium intakes are lower, the main sources being cereals and sometimes the soft bones found in some fish. The absorption of calcium from the intestine is closely regulated and depends on vitamin D, but also the availability of dietary calcium. Some food substances form complexes or insoluble calcium salts that cannot be absorbed. The most important is phytic acid found in cereal bran and some nuts and pulses. When bread is leavened, the enzyme phytase in the yeast partially breaks down the phytate, improving the availability of calcium and other minerals. Populations that consume unleavened whole grain bread, such as chapatis and tortillas, absorb a lower amount of calcium and other minerals. The level of dietary protein and phosphorus can affect the metabolism of calcium as increased protein intakes reduce the reabsorption of calcium in the kidneys, whereas, high phosphorus intakes increase the reabsorption.

Rickets and osteoporosis are two health problems related to calcium metabolism. Calcium deficiency reduces the growth rate of children, but calcium deficiency alone does not seem to result in rickets, a condition in which bones fail to calcify properly and become distorted. However, it may contribute to rickets when vitamin D status is low. Nor does calcium deficiency seem to be the cause of osteoporosis, the progressive loss of bone density with age leading to brittle bones. The main causes are inactivity and the reduced levels of sex hormones in women after middle age. Bone reaches its maximum density (peak bone density) at about the age of 30 and a high density can protect from the effects of osteoporosis in later life. Therefore, adequate calcium and vitamin D intakes up to this age are important, but high intakes of calcium have no beneficial effect once the bone density has been achieved. In the UK, the main sources of calcium in the diet are milk and dairy products (48%), white bread (9%) and vegetables (7%) (Gregory *et al.*, 1990).

3.7.3.2 *Phosphorus*

Phosphorus is an essential component of the mineral structure of bones and teeth where it occurs in the ratio of 1 : 2 with calcium. Eighty-five percent of the phosphorus in the adult body is in the bone, the remainder occurs in soft tissues where it plays an important role in many chemical reactions as a phosphate ion in lipids, proteins, carbohydrates, nucleic acid and enzymes. Energy for metabolic processes is derived mainly from the phosphate bonds of such compounds as adenosine triphosphate (ATP) and creatine phosphate.

Phosphorus occurs in almost all foods, the major contributors being protein rich foods and cereal grains. Food additives used in processing also contribute. The precise requirement for phosphorus is not known, but allowances set in various countries recommend quantities approximately equal to calcium. Dietary deficiency is rare except in premature infants fed human milk exclusively, or in people using the antacid aluminium hydroxide for long periods which binds phosphorus, making it unavailable. Deficiency results in bone mineral loss, weakness, anorexia, malaise and pain. Relative excess of phosphorus where dietary calcium is low and the calcium:phosphorus ratio is less than 1 : 2 has been shown to lower blood calcium levels. Meats, and fish without bones, contain 15–20 times more phosphorus than calcium; eggs, grains, nuts and legumes contain only twice the amount. Only milk products and green leafy vegetables contain more calcium than phosphorus.

3.7.3.3 *Magnesium*

The adult body contains 20–30 g magnesium of which approximately 40% is in the muscles and soft tissues, 1% in the extracellular fluid and almost 60% in the skeleton. Plasma magnesium levels remain constant by homeostatic mechanisms. Magnesium is involved in many biochemical processes including all biosynthetic processes, glycolysis, formation of cyclic-AMP, membrane transport and transmission of the genetic code. More than 300 enzymes are activated by magnesium. Intracellular magnesium controls cellular metabolism and extracellular magnesium, along with calcium, is critical in nerve and muscular function. Magnesium depletion can occur in gastrointestinal disease with malabsorption or excessive fluid losses, with deficient intravenous or intragastric feeding, or with drugs that interfere with magnesium conservation, as well as in general malnutrition and alcoholism; purely dietary deficiency has not been reported. Unprocessed foods all contain magnesium, with high concentrations in nuts, legumes and grains, but most is removed in the milling of grains. Magnesium is present in chlorophyll and so green vegetables are another good source. Animal products and fruit, with the exception of bananas, are relatively poor sources. Diets high in unrefined grains and in vegetables are much higher in magnesium than refined diets with considerable quantities of meat and dairy products.

3.7.4 Trace elements

3.7.4.1 *Fluoride*

Although fluoride is not classed as an essential nutrient, it has such a dramatic effect on the incidence and prevalence of dental decay, that dental caries could be considered a fluoride deficiency disease. Where water is not naturally or artificially fluoridated, the main dietary sources are tea and fish (if the soft bones are eaten). Variable amounts may also be inadvertently ingested from fortified sources such as toothpaste and mouthwash as well as advertently from fluoride tablets or drops. Despite the effectiveness of fluoride only a small proportion of the water supply in the UK is fluoridated. Opposition to fluoridation in the UK and the US is based on fears of 'unnatural' additions to water, overdosing, and unfounded claims of connections with cancer. On the basis of accumulated evidence of its beneficial effects fluoridation has been endorsed in the US by the National Institute of Dental Research, the American Medical Association, the National Cancer Institute, and the National Nutrition Consortium. In the UK, it has been endorsed by the British Dental Association, the Royal College of Physicians and the British Medical Association among other authoritative bodies.

3.7.4.2 *Iron*

Iron is a constituent of the functional compounds haemoglobin, myoglobin, and several enzymes. In addition, up to 30% of the iron in the body is in storage forms such as ferritin and haemosiderin in the spleen, liver and bone marrow, and a small amount attached to the blood transport protein transferrin. Body iron content is regulated through changes in intestinal absorption, influenced by body stores, the chemical nature of iron in the food, and concomitant dietary factors that increase or inhibit absorption. Iron is widely distributed in food, and in the UK cereal products provide 42% of the dietary iron, while meat and meat products provide 23% and vegetables 15% (Gregory et al., 1990). Dietary supplements provide 2% of average total iron intakes for men, and 15% for women. Iron in the form of haem in meat is better absorbed than the inorganic, non-haem iron in plant foods. Absorption of non-haem iron is facilitated by vitamin C and other organic acids if consumed at the same time, as well as by some proteins, but it is hindered by other food components including phytate, dietary fibre, calcium and tea. Iron deficiency which leads to anaemia is mainly due to a loss of blood at a rate greater than it can be replaced by absorption from the diet, as a result of intestinal parasites especially hookworm, or heavy menstrual losses. Iron deficiency anaemia is particularly common in women, but also occurs in the UK in infants and young children, especially in Asian communities (BNF, 1995).

3.7.4.3 *Zinc*

Zinc deficiency resulting in impaired growth and sexual development has been identified in population groups in the Middle East, who consume diets low in rich sources of zinc such as meat, and high in phytates found in unleavened bread.

It may exist in other communities where the staple food is chapatis or tortillas, and may partially account for the reduced stature of such populations. Zinc is implicated in immune function and therefore resistance to disease.

3.7.4.4 *Selenium*

Selenium is essential for at least two oxidase enzymes, including the antioxidant enzyme glutathione peroxidase, which enhances the ability of cells to cope with oxidative stress. Intakes vary widely according to the selenium content of the soil on which the foods were grown. Selenium deficiency may contribute to various degenerative diseases including cancer, although a firm link has not been established. Excess selenium results in dermatitis, abnormal nails, brittle hair and neurological abnormalities, and some studies show that areas of high selenium may be related to a higher prevalence of dental caries.

3.7.4.5 *Strontium*

Strontium can replace calcium in tooth enamel, and there is an inverse relationship with dental caries. Radioactive strontium in the fall-out of nuclear explosions contaminates crops and pasture in the affected area, and may be incorporated in the food supply. The absorption, storage and excretion of strontium is similar to that of calcium, and so is concentrated in the milk of animals and in bones and teeth. The adjacent bone marrow is therefore susceptible to damage by radiation.

3.7.4.6 *Lithium*

Lithium is not an essential nutrient, but it is effective as a pharmacological agent in manic depressive disease. An inverse relationship between lithium levels and dental caries has been observed.

Table 3.1 Consumption for selected foods, by region, 1996 (grams per person per week)

Consumption	England	Wales	Scotland	N. Ireland
Milk and cream (ml)	2094	2153	2181	2114
Cheese	112	107	108	73
Carcase meat	243	241	213	289
Other meat and meat products	698	729	729	702
Fish	155	147	151	131
Eggs (no.)	1.87	1.80	1.99	2.19
Fats and oils	229	226	209	261
Sugar and preserves	184	200	179	189
Vegetables	2141	2153	1899	2422
of which:				
fresh potatoes	810	862	725	1327
fresh green vegetables	242	221	159	182
other fresh vegetables	498	456	433	400
processed vegetables	591	614	582	513
Fruit	1035	1038	900	702
Bread	740	798	830	952
Other Cereals	824	738	709	835
Beverages	65	65	58	49
Soft drinks (ml)				
Alcoholic drinks (ml)	1422	1500	1515	1770
Confectionery	384	357	425	144
	58	72	55	46

3.7.4.7 *Molybdenum*

Molybdenum plays a role in several enzymes. Its concentration in foods varies considerably depending on where the food was grown, the main contributions to the diet being from milk, pulses and cereals. Deficiencies have been reported only in long term total parenteral nutrition and in rare inborn errors of metabolism, but toxicity can be a problem in animals and in humans where high environmental levels exist, as it antagonises metabolism of the essential element copper. There is some evidence that molybdenum is cariostatic.

3.8 OTHER BIOLOGICALLY ACTIVE SUBSTANCES

Apart from nutrients and dietary fibre, food contains a wide range of substances that are biologically active. Little scientific attention has been paid to possible functions in the past, but recently there has been extensive research into their protective effects against some common degenerative diseases. These include various antioxidants that reduce the rate of oxidation of susceptible substances, such as polyunsaturated fatty acids, by neutralising free radicals, highly reactive molecules that increase the rate of aging, and of the development of degenerative diseases including heart disease, cataracts and cancers. Non-nutrient antioxidants in food include: ubiquinone (coenzyme Q) and phenolic compounds, for example, phytoestrogens, flavonoids and phenolic acids. The food preservative chemicals butylated hydroxytoluene (BHT) and butylated hydroxyanisole (BHA) are also antioxidants, and are likely to have a physiological role.

3.9 DIETARY PATTERNS

In poor countries, carbohydrate, mainly starch, provides up to 80% of energy intakes, whereas, in the richer countries of North America, Europe

Table 3.2 Consumption for selected foods by income group, 1996 (grams per person per week)

| Consumption | Income group* | | | | | |
| | Households with one or more earners | | | | Households without an earner | |
	A	B	C	D	E1	E2
Milk and cream (ml)	1967	1964	2058	2123	2468	2192
Cheese	127	119	111	91	118	90
Meat and meat products	887	904	950	958	978	951
Fish	164	136	139	139	213	156
Eggs (no.)	1.62	1.56	1.80	1.98	2.22	2.26
Fats and oils	184	190	223	249	283	238
Sugar and preserves	103	130	166	204	264	267
Fruit	1348	1070	883	795	1422	781
Vegetables	1999	1948	2075	2171	2630	2198
of which:						
fresh potatoes	625	664	818	871	1093	920
fresh green vegetables	253	211	211	193	340	197
other fresh vegetables	588	487	432	429	690	412
processed vegetables	533	586	614	678	507	669
Cereals (including bread)	1441	1485	1598	1514	1635	1544
Beverages	56	53	57	64	83	78
Soft drinks (ml)	979	922	964	888	758	832
Alcoholic drinks (ml)	538	457	379	228	481	221
Confectionery	63	62	56	48	66	48

* Definition by the gross weekly income of the head of household:
  A, £595 and over.
  B, £310 and under £595.
  C, £150 and under £310.
  D, under £150.
  E1, £150 and over.
  E2, under £150.
Source: MAFF (1997). © Crown Copyright. Reproduced with permission: Controller of Her Majesty's Stationary Office.

and Australia, carbohydrates account for less than 50% of energy consumed, with up to half coming from sugars.

Food consumption and preferences are moulded by many geographic, economic and social factors, but certain trends can be discerned internationally. As people become more affluent they change their consumption away from coarse grain cereals such as millet and sorghum to wheat and rice, and then increasingly replace cereal and root crop staples with animal products, especially meat. Other additions to the diet are refined sugar and more expensive fruits and processed foods.

These changes in types of food consumed result in progressive changes in the proportion of energy coming from each nutrient constituent. The percentage of energy from protein is

Table 3.3 Nutritional value of household food by region, 1996

	England	Wales	Scotland	N. Ireland
	Intake per person per day			
Energy (kcal)	1860	1860	1810	1960
(MJ)	7.8	7.8	7.6	8.2
Total protein (g)	65.0	65.2	64.7	67.5
Animal protein (g)	39.7	40.1	40.1	40.1
Fat (g)	82	82	80	87
Fatty acids:				
saturated (g)	31.6	32.0	31.7	35.0
monounsaturated (g)	29.4	29.1	29.0	30.5
polyunsaturated (g)	14.9	14.8	13.8	15.0
Cholesterol (mg)	233	231	232	255
Carbohydrate (g)	229	230	220	242
of which:				
total sugars (g)	92	96	89	90
non-milk extrinsic sugars (g)	53	56	50	51
starch (g)	137	134	131	153
Fibre (as NSP) (g)	12.5	12.3	11.6	13.1
Calcium (mg)	820	814	825	800
Iron (mg)	10.1	10.0	10.0	10.7
Zinc (mg)	7.8	7.8	7.8	8.0
Magnesium (mg)	230	229	223	230
Sodium (g)	2.59	2.69	2.77	2.84
Potassium (g)	2.61	2.64	2.53	2.62
Thiamin (mg)	1.44	1.47	1.41	1.58
Riboflavin (mg)	1.60	1.60	1.58	1.62
Niacin equivalent (mg)	26.5	26.6	26.0	27.4
Vitamin B_6 (mg)	2.0	2.0	1.9	2.2
Vitamin B_{12} (μg)	4.3	4.2	4.4	4.1
Folate (μg)	250	243	234	259
Vitamin C (mg)	55	54	49	45
Vitamin A				
retinol (μg)	581	542	543	538
β-carotene (μg)	1700	1760	1480	1450
Total (retinol equivalent) (μg)	864	835	790	779
Vitamin D (μg)	3.37	3.44	3.14	3.40
Vitamin E (mg)	10.8	10.9	9.9	10.5
	Food energy* (%)			
Fat	39.7	39.6	40.1	39.9
of which:				
saturated fatty acids	15.3	15.5	15.8	16.1
Carbohydrate	46.3	46.3	45.6	46.4

* As a percentage of estimated average requirement.

Source: MAFF (1997). © Crown Copyright. Reproduced with permission: Controller of Her Majesty's Stationary Office.

fairly constant, between 10–15%, although with increasing affluence animal sources of protein increasingly replace vegetable sources. Differences in the percentage of energy from carbohydrate are therefore reflected by reciprocal differences in calories from fat. Poor countries may have only 10% of the calories coming from fat, while many of the rich have approximately 40%.

A high proportion of energy from fat is implicated in heart disease, obesity and some cancers. Dietary guidelines in most affluent countries recommend reducing fat intake to approximately 30–35% of the calories, and increasing carbohydrates to approximately 55%, (while limiting extracted sugar to no more than 10%). In contrast, the very low levels of fat in the diets of some poor countries can be problematic for the consumption of adequate energy, particularly in children.

These general patterns describe food consumption under normal circumstances. In times of food shortage, plants that are not normally part of the diet, or that may even be toxic may be consumed. These famine foods can include coarse grains, root crops resistant to drought and other environmental disasters, various wild plants, tulip bulbs and even ground date stones. In some cases such foods are nutritionally sound, but carry a social stigma, as they are not preferred by taste or custom, and are associated with poverty and distress.

3.9.1 Dietary patterns in the UK

Even within the UK there is considerable variation in food and nutrient consumption as shown in the annual National Food Surveys and Family Expenditure Surveys, and the Diet and Nutrition Surveys of particular age groups. These all show regional, socioeconomic, age and sex differences in consumption. Time trends can be seen by comparison of annual surveys.

An example from the 1996 National Food Survey of variation in household food consumption by region is shown in Table 3.1, and by income group in Table 3.2 (MAFF, 1997). Table 3.3 shows the corresponding nutritional values (MAFF, 1997). From Table 3.1, it can be seen that in Scotland there is a lower consumption of carcase meat, fats and oils, sugar and preserves, vegetables, fruit and confectionery eaten at home than in England and Wales, but there is a higher consumption of meat products and soft drinks. This translates into a lower intake of total energy and all nutrients, however, the percentage of total energy from fat and saturates is slightly higher (Table 3.3). Foods eaten outside the home constitute 12% on average of the total energy consumed in the UK, alcohol being a major component consumed outside the home (MAFF, 1997).

In the lower income groups, consumption of cheese, fruit, soft drinks, alcoholic drinks and confectionery is lower and that of milk, meat products, eggs, fats and oils, sugar and preserves, vegetables, cereals and beverages is higher than the higher income groups (Table 3.2). Food eaten outside the home also varies by income group. In terms of nutrient intakes, the low income groups have higher intakes of energy and all macronutrients, and a slightly higher percent energy from fat. Lower socioeconomic groups also have higher intakes of calcium, retinol and vitamin D, but lower intakes of vitamin C and β-carotene (MAFF, 1997).

Table 3.4 Contribution of main food types to average daily intakes of protein, fat, carbohydrate and sugars in the British diet

	Protein (%)	Fat (%)	Carbohydrate (%)	Sugars (%)
Cereal products	23	19	46	23
Milk products	17	15	6	13
Eggs and egg dishes	4	4	0	0
Fat spreads	0	16	0	0
Meat and products	36	24	5	1
Fish and fish dishes	6	3	1	0
Vegetables	9	11	16	6
Fruit and nuts	1	1	4	8
Sugar, confectionery and preserves	1	3	13	29
Beverages	1	0	7	17
Miscellaneous	2	3	3	3

Source: Gregory *et al.* (1990). © Crown Copyright. Reproduced with permission: Office for National Statistics.

The Dietary and Nutritional Survey of British Adults shows that protein provides 15% of the total energy in the average diet (Gregory *et al.*, 1990). Fats provided 38% and carbohydrate provided 42% of total energy intakes, with total sugars providing about 20% of total energy intakes. The main food sources of these macronutrients are shown in Table 3.4.

4

DENTAL CARIES – AETIOLOGY AND PATHOGENENSIS

4.1 INTRODUCTION

Together with the common cold, dental caries is perhaps the most prevalent disease of modern man, but unlike the cold, its effects leave behind defects that are permanent. While recent decreases in the prevalence of caries in children in the UK have revolutionised the perception of caries and its control, there is still a long way to go in controlling the disease, even in children. Indeed, prolongation of the life of the dentition into old age leads to increased opportunities for carious attacks, for example, caries of the exposed roots of teeth following gum recession. The sequelae of caries in terms of morbidity and cost to the nation are still among the highest for any disease. It is essential, therefore, to continue to expand our understanding of the causes and pathology of caries as a basis for further advances in the prevention of the disease.

'Dental caries' literally means 'tooth rot', and is a descriptive term applied to a condition or group of conditions in which the dental hard tissues are progressively broken down leading, if unopposed, to infection and death of the pulp. The process of caries first involves dissolution of the mineral phase of the tooth surface by organic acids formed by the bacterial fermentation of sugars derived from the diet. The bacteria are attached to tooth surfaces sheltered from the forces of mastication or brushing as a sticky, almost invisible film called *dental plaque*. The presence of saliva, on the other hand, plays a key role in the control of the disease over a period of time. Once the sugars are cleared from the mouth, the diffusion of saliva into the plaque raises the pH at the tooth surface and the carious process stops. If no more sugar enters the plaque for a considerable period of time, the saliva can repair the initial damage caused. This process distinguishes caries from dental erosion, which is due to the direct action of acids, including food acids, on the hard tissues without the involvement of plaque bacteria. Later stages

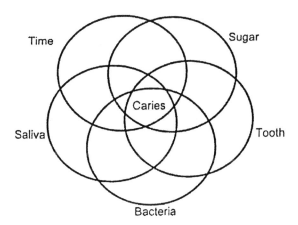

Figure 4.1 The inter-relationship of five factors in the production of dental caries.

of caries, once the process has reached the dentine, involve a more complex pathology including bacterial breakdown of the organic framework of the tissue.

The aetiology of caries involves five major factors: teeth, saliva, bacteria in plaque, dietary sugars and time (Figure 4.1). All of this can be influenced by the social, cultural, geographical and economic environments in which the affected individual and community exist.

4.1.1 The tooth

The dissolution of the mineral salts of the tooth (hydroxyapatite) proceeds according to the formula:

$$Ca_{10}(PO_4)_6(OH)_2 + 8H^+ \leftrightarrows 10Ca^{2+} + 6HPO_4^{2-} + 2H_2O$$

The rate of dissolution, or *demineralisation*, will be affected by the concentration of hydrogen ions (pH) at the tooth surface which will increase demineralisation, and of calcium and phosphate ions derived from saliva which will oppose it. Calcium and phosphate ions at the tooth surface are in dynamic equilibrium with those in the plaque overlaying it. At normal levels of pH at the tooth surface the levels of calcium and phosphate ions around the teeth are such that no demineralisation occurs, in fact, the equilibrium favours passage of ions into the surface; that is, the aqueous environment at the tooth surface is 'super-saturated' with respect to hydroxyapatite. However, as the hydrogen ion concentration rises (and thus the pH falls), an equilibrium point is reached when the levels of calcium and phosphate ions can no longer prevent demineralisation. This equilibrium point is called the *critical pH*; it is higher for dentine than enamel. When the plaque pH is above the critical level, the concentrations of calcium and phosphate in the plaque are by definition sufficient to prevent demineralisation. However, when the plaque pH is below the critical level the net reaction will be loss of mineral from the tooth. Because the dissolution reaction above is reversible, this implies that crystals of hydroxyapatite can regrow (be repaired) after an episode of acid dissolution, a process known as *remineralisation*. There is good evidence that caries occurs only when the balance of dissolution and repair is tipped towards excess dissolution, that is, when demineralisation exceeds remineralisation. This balance of the two factors has been called the 'ionic seesaw' (Figure 4.2).

The ionic seesaw can be tilted towards dental health by increasing the calcium and phosphate levels at the tooth surface principally through access of saliva, thus lowering the critical pH and requiring a bigger pH drop to cause demineralisation. In addition, the presence of fluoride ions at the tooth surface or inside developing caries will favour remineralisation. This is because fluoride can replace hydroxyl groups in hydroxyapatite to form fluorapatite:

$$Ca_{10}(PO_4)_6(OH_2) + 2F \rightarrow Ca_{10}(PO_4)_6F_2 + 2OH$$

Fluorapatite is more stable than hydroxyapatite which means it is both less soluble and more likely to form when remineralisation takes place in the presence of fluoride. The remineralised enamel may thus be less soluble and, therefore, more resistant to subsequent attack than the initial sound enamel.

Thus, the carious process consists of innumerable separate incidents when the plaque pH falls below the critical value, each incident usually occurring over a period of between 20–60 minutes depending on a number of factors, such as the nature of the food and the quality and quantity of the saliva. The demineralisation first occurs just below the surface of the enamel leaving the surface intact. This permits repair to take place under favourable conditions, retaining the integrity of the dental tissues. However, if the cariogenic challenge is too great, the balance of the ionic seesaw is tilted towards mineral loss and eventually the enamel surface collapses causing permanent damage that cannot be reversed. This can occur rapidly over a period of a few months, but more usually it is a slow process that may take several years to occur. The process occurs more rapidly on exposed root surfaces than on enamel surfaces as the former are less mineralised.

4.1.2 Saliva

It is clear from this description of the carious process that the presence and composition of the saliva is crucial to the health of the dentition. Its chemical composition, buffering capacity and quantity all play an important role in combating caries. It is also important for saliva to gain easy

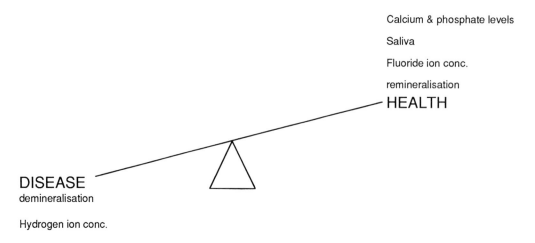

Calcium & phosphate levels

Saliva

Fluoride ion conc.

remineralisation

HEALTH

DISEASE
demineralisation

Hydrogen ion conc.

Figure 4.2 The influence of the ionic seesaw on the health of the dentition.

access to the plaque under which the carious process is taking place, so that it can quickly restore the pH to levels above the critical value and to repair the minute amount of damage that may have occurred. The tooth surfaces to which saliva cannot penetrate easily (e.g. deep pits and fissures; surfaces in contact with adjacent teeth) are more susceptible to caries than those with free access to saliva.

4.1.3 Bacteria in plaque

The main concentration of bacteria in the mouth resides in the dental plaque and constitutes most of the plaque volume. There are many species of bacteria in plaque that can ferment sugars, but only a few are capable of doing this once the critical pH has been reached. The main groups involved in this are the mutans streptococci (*S. mutans* and *S. sobrinus*) and lactobacilli. The crucial role of bacteria in caries was demonstrated when caries-susceptible rats born and raised in sterile environments, failed to develop caries when fed a high sugar, cariogenic diet. However, when individual bacterial species were introduced into their mouths under carefully controlled conditions, variable amounts of caries were produced demonstrating that different species possessed different abilities to induce caries.

Dietary sugars

Bacteria utilise dietary sugars—glucose, fructose, galactose, sucrose, maltose, lactose—very efficiently, although lactose and galactose are fermented only slowly. Bacterial and salivary enzymes (amylases) can also break down starch to maltose and maltotriose contributing to acid production, but this proceeds more slowly such that the buffering capacity of saliva has time to influence the process, often preventing the critical pH from being reached.

The principal way in which bacteria use sugars to produce acid is via the glycolytic sequence of linked enzyme reactions. This sequence starts with a molecule of glucose which is transported via a permease into the bacterial cell. Here it is phosphorylated and catabolised to produce energy and primarily lactic, but also acetic, succinic and proprionic acids. Under conditions of low glucose, the sugar is transported via a specific transport system (phosphoenolpyruvate transferase system) and the major metabolic end products produced by the bacteria are ethanol, formate and acetate. At the same time, energy is released for the requirements of the bacteria including their growth. Sugars other than glucose are mostly converted to glucose inside the bacterial cell, to enter the glycolytic sequence (Figure 4.3).

Acids such as lactic acid give rise to hydrogen ions when they dissociate:

$$CH_3CHOH.COOH \rightarrow CH_3CHOH.COO + H^+ \text{ (acid)}$$
(lactic acid) (lactic anion)

Increasing concentrations of hydrogen ions are measured as a fall in pH, and have the consequence of increasing the solubility of the mineral phase of the teeth, as already described.

If the hydrogen ion concentration is very low, lactate anions may act as hydrogen ion acceptors or buffers. The point at which the number of acid molecules and lactic anions are exactly equal is called the dissociation constant and is usually defined in terms of the pH ('pK'). Above the pK, acids will tend to dissociate while below the pK the anion will accept a hydrogen ion. If the pK of an acid:anion pair is around that found in plaque, then it may function as a buffer and help to prevent a fall in pH by 'mopping up' hydrogen ions. Acid:anion systems with suitable pKs include $H_2PO_4 : HPO_4$ and $H_2CO_3 : HCO_3$. These two systems are present in saliva and constitute very important factors controlling pH changes in plaque. Buffers are also present in foods which may modify the plaque pH response.

The formation of acid from dietary sugars thus occurs in close proximity to the tooth surface, and the resulting changes in pH in the plaque can be followed to gain insight into the caries process and the effect of various factors on it. The characteristic form of the pH response in plaque to sugar, plotted against time, is called the *Stephan Curve* (Figure 4.4).

Acid production is very rapid with a minimum pH being found 5–10 minutes following exposure to sugars. The pH then slowly returns to the baseline value of between 6.5 and 7.0 owing to metabolism of the acids in plaque, neutralisation by salivary buffers and diffusion of the acids from the plaque into saliva.

The episodic nature of the Stephan Curve indicates that the frequency and duration of ingestion of dietary sugars is an important aspect in the aetiology of caries. It also demonstrates that anything that will lower the critical pH or will restore the pH quickly back to levels above the critical value will also be of benefit. In addition, is clear that food which lowers the plaque pH but fails to depress it below the critical value will play little if any role in the carious process.

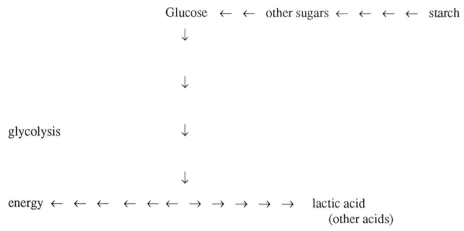

Figure 4.3 The breakdown of glucose to acids in the glycolytic sequence.

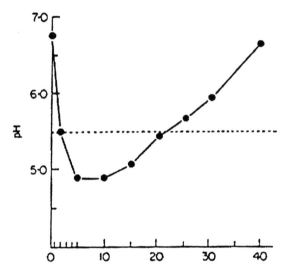

Figure 4.4 Stephan Curve of plaque pH vs time (mins) following use of a glucose solution as a mouthrinse. The calculated critical pH is indicated as a dotted line below which the tooth is under carious attack.

4.2 THE CARIOUS PROCESS

The first clinically detectable change in the tooth as the result of caries is the formation of an opaque 'white spot' on the otherwise translucent enamel due to an increase in porosity which in turn leads to increased light-scattering. This porosity is due to the loss of the more soluble elements of the enamel. As has already been mentioned, the porosity occurs some 10–20 μm below the surface, while the overlying enamel remains intact. The most reasonable explanation for the formation of a *subsurface lesion* is the remineralisation of initially damaged crystals in the superficial zone by calcium and phosphate ions diffusing outwards from the dissolving crystals in the subsurface layer. White-spot lesions are at least partially reversible if re-mineralising conditions supervene before the undermined surface layer collapses. These

lesions are defined by the area of overlying dental plaque so that at the gingival margin the lesion will have the shape of the contour of the gingival tissues.

For the lesion to occur it is most likely that the dental plaque will have been in place and undisturbed for a period in excess of 7–14 days during which time sufficient mineral will be lost from the subsurface of the enamel with the formation of a white-spot lesion.

If the carious process proceeds, the subsurface demineralisation becomes more marked and spreads towards the dentine, which may respond by laying down a protective layer of 'tertiary dentine' in an attempt to defend the vitality of the pulp. As the decay reaches the dentine, it spreads rapidly along the enamel-dentine junction. The loss of mineral in the enamel leads to the breakdown of the surface and the undermined enamel is lost. This is the stage at which an examining dentist will diagnose a cavity, and at which the patient may become aware of sensitivity to hot or cold foods and drinks or sweet or salty items which have a high osmotic pressure.

Once the bacteria reach the dentine they can pass down the dentinal tubules and continue to produce acid and demineralisation. Once the organic material is freed from mineral crystals, proteolytic enzymes from the bacteria break down the collagen fibres of the dentine. Eventually, if unchecked, the bacteria and their toxins reach the pulp causing an acute inflammation with associated severe throbbing pain. Soon the pulp dies and the inflammation spreads down the root canal into the tissues surrounding the apex of the tooth resulting in an apical abscess. The tooth is now extremely sensitive to biting or even touching and a swelling may result in the soft tissue overlying the adjacent bone. If the tooth is not extracted then technically difficult and time-consuming treatment will be required of the pulp chamber, root canal and periapical tissues.

4.2.1 Caries models

Because human caries is so complex and people so difficult to control, model experiments have been established which mimic certain aspects of the disease in an attempt to understand the process in more detail. These vary in sophistication and in the degree to which they reflect the factors influencing the pathology. They have been classified (American Dental Association, 1986) into *in vitro* models, animal experiments, *in situ* studies and *in vivo* trials.

In vitro models are biochemical experiments carried out in the laboratory. They can vary in their complexity, and are highly controllable to give repeatable results. However, they rarely reproduce more than one or two factors simultaneously, and do not resemble the real events of the disease as it occurs at the tooth-plaque interphase.

Examples of *in vitro* models (Clarkson, 1986) include:

● tests of enamel solubility in acidic buffers containing protective substances derived from foods;
● tests of acid production from carbohydrate foods with oral bacteria from, for example, saliva;
● a combination of the above—enamel solubility during incubation of saliva with foods;
● tests of enamel demineralisation in an 'artificial mouth' with an alternating supply of food and saliva to inoculated, extracted teeth to mimic the intermittent supply of substrate with meals and snacks.

Experimental animals have also been used in caries research. Again they may focus on only one or a few of the factors involved in caries, but are more realistic and, therefore, give more information which can be interpreted with more confidence as being relevant to caries in humans. The animal which may be nearest to the human in terms of the physiological and pathological processes controlling caries is the monkey. Although this species is usually too expensive to keep in any numbers, several useful experiments have been reported in the literature (Bowen, 1981). As dental caries can be produced under certain conditions in rats and hamsters, and because these animals are less expensive to keep, they have been used extensively in this

research. Caries in rats shares many similarities to that in man, although, among other things, differences due to the different nature of the dentitions and composition of saliva mean that findings cannot be directly transposed to humans. The level of control over the conditions under which rats live is much greater, of course, than with human subjects especially with regard to the oral microflora and the frequency with which a cariogenic diet is eaten. Animal feeding trials have long been used to study the influence of diet and nutrition on the carious process (Tanzer, 1986).

In situ models are carried out on human volunteers in place of expensive clinical trials which are difficult to control and in many cases impossible to conduct for ethical reasons. Experiments on human subjects are clearly preferable for the greater validity which they give to the conclusions derived.

Examples of *in situ* models include:

● studies of plaque pH after eating a variety of carbohydrate foods indicating the acidogenicity of the food (Harper *et al.*, 1986);
● studies of de- and re-mineralisation of pieces of human or animal enamel cut from extracted teeth, sterilised and fixed in some device to volunteers' teeth (Manning and Edgar, 1992).

In vivo trials are more difficult to arrange principally for ethical reasons, and the results of small scale studies conducted under artificial circumstances on human volunteers are not yet acceptable to national regulatory bodies.

An example of an *in vivo* study is:

● the production of early, reversible carious lesions in the mouths of volunteers using frequent intakes of sugar containing mouthrinses over a 3-week period (von de Fehr, 1970).

The results of such model experiments have contributed to current advice concerning the selection of foods for the prevention of caries by individuals or by population groups. While the only conclusive way of demonstrating the validity of such dietary advice is by means of a randomised clinical trial, it is usually impossible or impractical to carry out such trials and we are forced to accept indirect evidence of the likely effect on caries of the consumption of individual foods.

Caries models have also been critical in the investigation of eating patterns, of the effects of saliva stimulation by foods and its interaction with caries, and of the efficacy of the anti-caries properties of fluoride and, more recently, xylitol.

4.2.2 Microbiology of dental caries

The survival of microorganisms at sites which are predisposed to becoming carious is associated with their ability to transport dietary sugars over a wide range of environmental conditions including a range of pH levels and sugar concentrations. Changes in plaque pH may be stressful and the ability to withstand prolonged and repeated exposure to low pH and the ability to metabolise carbohydrates to produce energy at low pH favour these microorganisms. Finally, the ability to synthesise extracellular polysaccharides (mutan, glucan and fructan) from sucrose facilitates the attachment of these bacteria to tooth surfaces and localises their fermentation products. In addition, the formation of intracellular polysaccharides as storage polymers from dietary sucrose and other sugars for use in the absence of dietary carbohydrates is also beneficial to these microorganisms. These characteristics are found in the lactobacilli, mutans streptococci and yeasts. A summary of the major interactions between dietary carbohydrates and dental plaque bacteria, principally streptococci, is shown in Figure 4.5. The microbial definition of a carious lesion is dependent, *inter alia*, on its location and severity.

4.2.3 The early carious lesion (white spot)

A selection of the microflora of the plaque overlying white-spot lesions and associated with the

immediate adjacent sound tooth surfaces was first studied by Duchin and van Houte (1978). They found that the proportion of mutans streptococci in the plaque overlying the lesion was significantly greater than in that on the surrounding sound tooth surface. The frequency of isolation of lactobacilli was low at both sites. These observations regarding the increased proportions of mutans streptococci in the plaque associated with the lesions were confirmed by Boyar *et al.* (1989), who studied a wider range of the plaque microflora associated with incipient caries in children. That lactobacilli may not contribute significantly to the initiation of caries was first reported by Hemmens *et al.* (1946). The frequency of isolation of these bacteria and their proportional representation in dental plaque increase after the formation of an overt carious cavity.

4.2.4 Nursing-bottle caries

The prolonged use of a feeding bottle containing a sugary liquid may result in the formation of a characteristic pattern of tooth decay with dental caries primarily limited to the upper and lower deciduous incisor teeth. This unfortunate situation arises if the sugar containing liquid is held in the mouth for considerable lengths of time, such as when asleep, or when drinks are consumed continuously for long periods while awake. In both instances the dental plaque microflora has access for long periods to suitable substrate for acid production and, as a consequence, a particularly rapid and characteristic form of tooth decay is initiated. Case reports of

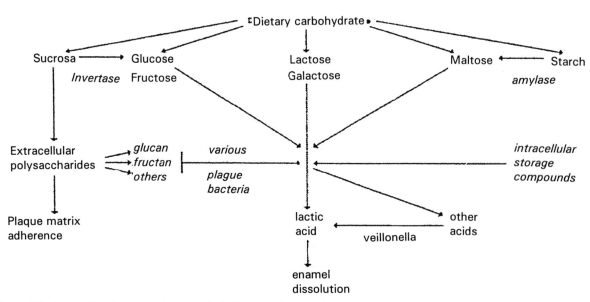

Figure 4.5 Interactions between dietary carbohydrates and plaque bacteria.
Source: Marsh and Martin (1992).

nursing caries have also been published where the authors claim that the condition has arisen from prolonged 'on-demand' breast-feeding, especially at night when the baby has fallen asleep with the teat still in its mouth.

The microflora of nursing-bottle caries have been reported by Milnes and Bowden (1985), who conducted a longitudinal study of two caries susceptible sites on the incisor teeth of infants initially aged between 10–16 months. Samples of plaque associated with white-spot lesions, frank cavities and caries-free surfaces in the caries-active children, and caries-free surfaces in the caries-free children were analysed for mutans streptococci, lactobacilli, actinomyces and veillonella. The plaque sample from the caries-free children had significantly lower levels of mutans streptococci (5.7%) and lactobacilli (0.01%) than sites from the caries-active children. However, there were no statistically significant differences between the levels of mutans streptococci and lactobacilli from the three different sites in the caries-active children.

The proportions of actinomyces and veillonella were not significantly altered by the onset of nursing-bottle caries, and were not significantly different between the two groups of children. The microflora of children who present with nursing caries is characterised by unusually high levels of both mutans streptococci and lactobacilli on both carious and apparently sound surfaces. Nonetheless, these observations further support a central role for mutans streptococci in the initiation of dental caries.

4.2.5 Coronal caries

Caries on the enamel of the crowns of the teeth is referred to as coronal caries, and occurs primarily on the occlusal surface of teeth and on the approximal surfaces in contact with the adjacent teeth. Coronal caries is the most prevalent of all types of caries and requires the greatest use of dental resources for its treatment. Longitudinal studies of the microflora associated with coronal caries have been restricted only to selected components of the flora. One reason for this is the sheer cost and logistics of studying the entire microflora of a large number of healthy tooth sites, only some of which will become carious. A second reason is the lack of media to support the growth of all the bacteria which might be present. A third is the continuous changes in the taxonomic status of those microorganisms which might be associated with the carious process, but whose involvement cannot be ascertained unless they can be accurately and reliably identified. The taxa most involved in the

caries process and which have undergone significant revisions in the last few years are the streptococci (Kilian et al., 1989; Beighton et al., 1991a), the actinomyces (Johnson et al., 1989) and the lactobacilli (Schleifer and Ludwid, 1996; Dicks et al., 1996).

The principal dental plaque microorganisms which have been studied in terms of their role in coronal caries have been the mutans streptococci, lactobacilli, 'Streptococcus sanguis', 'Streptococcus mitis' and Actinomyces spp. However, the proportions of these taxa vary greatly and even when present they rarely represent greater than 10–15% of the total flora. Routinely they are isolated using selective culture media. From the many longitudinal studies it is clear than only the mutans streptococci and lactobacilli are associated with dental caries on the occlusal surfaces and approximal sites.

Hardie et al. (1977) investigated the proportions of mutans streptococci and lactobacilli in successive samples taken from interproximal spaces before and after the diagnosis of dental caries. They found that the proportion of mutans streptococci increased just before the clinical diagnosis of dental caries, rose abruptly during the period of lesion initiation, continued to rise for 3–4 months and then declined. In contrast, the proportion of lactobacilli remained low and relatively constant until after the diagnosis of dental caries. The microflora of occlusal fissures before and after the diagnosis of dental caries were studied by Ikeda et al. (1973) and Loesche and Straffon (1979). Their observations were similar to those of Hardie et al. (1977) except that the initiation of dental caries tended to be preceded by elevated levels of both mutans streptococci and lactobacilli. Loesche and Straffon (1979) undertook a bacteriological analysis on 195 teeth that received four examinations at intervals of approximately every six months. The data obtained from 42 carious and 153 caries-free fissures indicated a role for S. mutans in the initiation of caries in most of these. The proportion of S. mutans increased significantly at the time of caries diagnosis and, by cross-sectional comparisons, it was demonstrated that the proportion of S. mutans in the carious fissures were significantly higher than in caries-free fissures. However, three subjects, who had a low caries experience, developed five new carious fissure lesions and in these, lactobacilli were the prominent members of the flora. Although the results implicated S. mutans in fissure decay, they showed that clinical decay could occur in a few instances in the absence of detectable S. mutans.

4.2.6 Occult caries

Occult caries is a recently recognised phenomenon in which occlusal surfaces appear to be clinically intact, but have a marked radiolucency in the dentine when examined using radiographs. It is suggested that the widespread use of fluoride toothpastes and other factors have reduced the rate of caries development in the enamel, so that it remains intact even when undermined by caries in the dentine. However, a recent study using data collected in 1968/1969 from 15-year-old people taking part in the Dutch longitudinal epidemiological Tiel/Culemborg fluoridation study, examined the influence of water fluoridation on the occurrence of occult caries. The 250 participants in Tiel, who received optimally fluoridated drinking water continuously from birth, had a mean of 2.54 clinically sound occlusal surfaces in first and second molars, of which bite-wing radiographs detected 0.43 surfaces (16.9%) with a radiolucency into dentine. The 245 participants in Culemborg who received water with a low concentration of fluoride (0.1 ppm F) had a mean 0.65 surfaces judged sound of which 0.16 (24.6%) showed a radiolucency into dentine. The results showed a proportional reduction of surfaces with occult caries in the fluoridated area compared to the control (Weerheijm *et al.*, 1997). This showed that occult caries is not a new phenomenon.

A recent study has reported the bacterial composition of carious dentine from 10 occult caries lesions and 17 small open lesions in children aged 8–18 years (de Soet *et al.*, 1995). *Actinomyces* spp., mutans streptococci, *S. sanguis*, *S. oralis*, *S. gordonii*, *S. mitis* and *Lactobacillus* spp. were isolated and *S. mutans* was found more often in the occult caries group. However, proportions of mutans streptococci were lower in the open lesion group and lactobacilli and *Actinomyces* spp. were found at similar levels in both groups. A more diverse range of streptococcal species and veillonella was found in the open lesion group, indicating a less complex microflora in occult caries, which in turn suggests that the aetiology of occult caries might be different from that of open caries.

4.2.7 Root-surface caries

Root caries occurs on the exposed roots of teeth and, although it may be diagnosed in adults of any age, it is mainly reported in the elderly. The lesions apparently initiate at the gingival margin where dental plaque has accumulated due to poor oral hygiene (Beighton *et al.*, 1991b). In

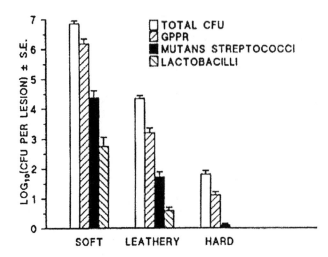

Figure 4.6 Comparison of the number of bacteria recovered from root-caries lesions classified according to texture.
Source: Beighton *et al.* (1993). Reproduced with permission: Journal of Dental Research.

longitudinal studies it has been shown that root surface sites from which mutans streptococci and lactobacilli were isolated are those most likely to become carious. Similar evidence does not support a role for *Actinomyces* spp. in the initiation of root caries (Ellen *et al.*, 1985). The microflora of root caries has been studied recently by several investigators (Bowden *et al.*, 1990; Bowden, 1990; van Houte *et al.*, 1994, 1996; Schupbach *et al.*, 1995). However, these studies are not comparable and the results are difficult to interpret. Different criteria were used to assess the clinical severity of the lesions sampled. In addition, methods were employed which did not sample discreetly from the infected dentine but rather from the overlying plaque with, or without, the underlying infected dentine.

It is possible to overcome these last two problems by the simple procedure of removing plaque from above the root-caries lesions with a sterile toothbrush (Beighton *et al.*, 1993) and using the criteria of Nyvad and Fejerskov (1985) to determine the clinical severity (soft, leathery or hard) of the lesion. Using this combined approach it has been possible to demonstrate that lesions classified as described above are microbiologically quite distinct (Beighton *et al.*, 1993) (Figure 4.6).

In keeping with the idea of the role of mutans streptococci and lactobacilli in the caries process, it has been demonstrated that the more severe and intrusive the perceived treatment needs of the lesions, the greater is the frequency of isolation of mutans streptococci and lactobacilli (Figure 4.7).

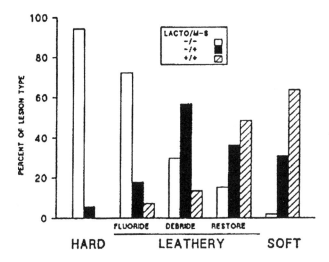

Figure 4.7 Frequency of isolation of mutans streptoccoci and lactobacilli from root-caries lesions classified according to treatment need.
Source: Beighton *et al.* (1993). Reproduced with permission: Journal of Dental Research.

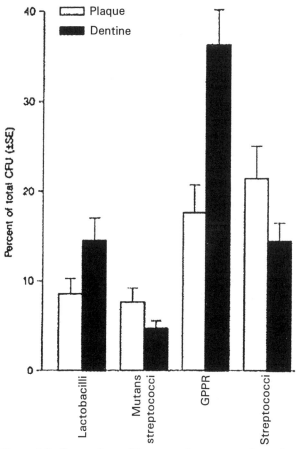

Figure 4.8 Comparison of the precentage composition of the microflora of plaque and dentine association with root-caries lesions.
Source: Beighton and Lynch (1995). Reproduced with permission: S. Karger AG, Basel.

There is evidence that the actinomyces are involved in the progression of root-carieslesions, as within the infected dentine the proportions of Gram-positive rods increase while those of mutans streptococci decrease (Beighton and Lynch, 1995) (Figure 4.8). The reasons why these bacteria are involved in the progression of caries may be related to their particular nutritional requirements and their relative fluoride resistance.

4.2.8 Role of non-mutans streptococci in dental caries

In the previous sections, there has been considerable emphasis on the role of mutans streptococci in the caries process. This arises from the many specific studies which have addressed the particular role of mutans streptococci to the exclusion of other streptococci. In both coronal and root-surface caries, it has been suggested that those streptococci ('low pH non-mutans streptococci') which produce large amounts of acid (pH < 4.2 in broth) may contribute significantly to the caries process (van Houte *et al.*, 1991, 1996; Sansone *et al.*, 1993). In most studies, these streptococci (*S. gordonii*, *S. oralis*, *S. mitis* and *S. anginosus*) outnumber the mutans streptococci, and because of this it has been suggested that they may play a significant role in the caries process. However, these studies have also suggested that a selection for non-mutans streptococci with an increased ability to grow at low pH occurs within the lesions (Table 4.1). Clearly, this microbial aspect of the initiation and progression of dental caries requires further investigation, and also highlights the polymicrobial nature of the bacterial popula-

tions involved in the loss of mineral from tooth tissues.

4.2.9 Effect of sugars on the oral microflora

The inclusion of sugars, especially sucrose, in the diet is associated with increased levels of dental caries. In the preceding sections, it has also been shown that the plaque and salivary levels of mutans streptococci, lactobacilli and yeasts are positively associated with the levels of dental caries. Attempts to complete this triangle of association by demonstrating that the presence of sugar in the diet significantly affects the levels of individual members of the oral microflora, have not been successful in people consuming their normal diet. For example, in a group of 328 12-year-old children, the levels of dental caries were significantly associated with the consumption of sugar (recorded using duplicate 3-day diet diaries plus interview), and with the salivary levels of both mutans streptococci and lactobacilli. However, there was no significant association between sugar consumption

Table 4.1 Comparison of the percentage distribution of lactobacilli, mutans streptococci, bifidibacterium and non-mutans streptococci, isolated from root caries lesions ($n = 84$) and sound tooth surfaces ($n = 223$) on the basis of their terminal pH values in 1% glucose broth

Organism	Terminal pH in 1% glucose broth					
	Advanced root-caries lesions			Sound root surfaces		
	<4.2	4.2–4.4	>4.4	<4.2	4.2–4.4	>4.4
Lactobacillus	100	0	0	0	0	0
Mutans streptococci	100	0	0	100	0	0
Bifidobacterium	68	11	21	0	0	0
Non-mutans streptococci	78	18	4	16	51	33

and the salivary levels of both mutans streptococci and lactobacilli (Beighton et al., 1996). These findings are similar to those from a variety of groups of Scandinavian children eating normal diets (Kristofferson and Birkhed, 1987; Stecksen-Blicks, 1987; Seppa et al.,1988). Another study found that the consumption of diets containing high levels of sucrose (115 g/day) compared to low levels (15 g/day), showed a non-significant three-fold increase in the proportions of mutans streptococci in plaque (Staat et al., 1975). However, no difference in the oral load of mutans streptococci was demonstrable between subjects consuming 0–3 or 8–12 between-meal sucrose eating events. Thus, increasing the sucrose content of the diet of individuals whose oral microflora contains commensal mutans streptococci does not significantly alter it. In monkeys harbouring undetectable levels of mutans streptococci, the introduction of a sucrose-containing diet rapidly increased the proportions of mutans streptococci so that within a few days after the sucrose was introduced the plaque levels were 10 times greater ($p < 0.001$) (Beighton et al., 1985).

In contrast to these studies, the reduction of sucrose from an average of 9.5 to 1.6 intakes of sugar per day for 6 weeks reduced significantly the number of mutans streptococci (S. mutans and S. sobrinus) and lactobacilli in saliva (Wennerholm et al., 1995) (Figure 4.9). However, no change in the proportion of mutans streptococci in the plaque of these subjects could be demonstrated. The removal of sucrose from the diet in two other studies also demonstrated significant two- to five-fold reductions in the oral load of mutans streptococci and lactobacilli (Kristoffersson and Birkhed, 1987; Andreen and Kohler, 1992).

4.2.10 The effect of sugar alcohols on the oral microflora

The sugar alcohols, xylitol and sorbitol, have been used in many studies as partial or complete substitutes for sucrose. The rationale for this is that dental plaque has a lower ability to produce acids rapidly from sugar alcohols compared to other sugars such as sucrose or fructose. Very few bacteria in dental plaque have the ability to utilise sorbitol for growth with the major exception of S. mutans, which will proliferate in the plaque of subjects consuming sorbitol-containing products.

Xylitol is transported into S. mutans via the fructose phosphenolpyruvate transferase system to form xylitol-5-phosphate. The consequence is that xylitol-5-phosphate is not catabolised by S. mutans and so inhibits the formation of more phosphoenolpyruvate from the transported carbohydrate. In addition, the phosphoenolpyruvate already formed has been used up in the transportation process (Waaler et al., 1985; Assev and Scheie, 1986). The combined effect is to kill the bacteria due to the intracellular accumulation of xylitol-5-phosphate and the depletion of phosphoenolpyruvate (Waaler et al., 1992). In use, the presence of xylitol in chewing gums and other foodstuffs reduces the oral levels of mutans streptococci (Loesche et al., 1984; Makinen et al., 1989) and, more especially, lowers the incidence of caries (Scheinin and Makinen, 1975; Figure 4.10).

4.2.11 Characteristics of foods which may modulate the caries attack

The type of food or drink in which fermentable carbohydrate is consumed will modulate the pH drop by virtue of its fundamental characteristics. In particular, it would be expected that sugar-containing dairy products would not produce a significant fall in the pH of plaque due to the considerable buffering capacity exerted by their combination of high levels of phosphate, protein and lipid. Thus up to 10% sucrose may be added to milk without a significant fall in pH being recorded. Consideration should also be given to the acidogenic potential of sugars added to, and

SALIVA

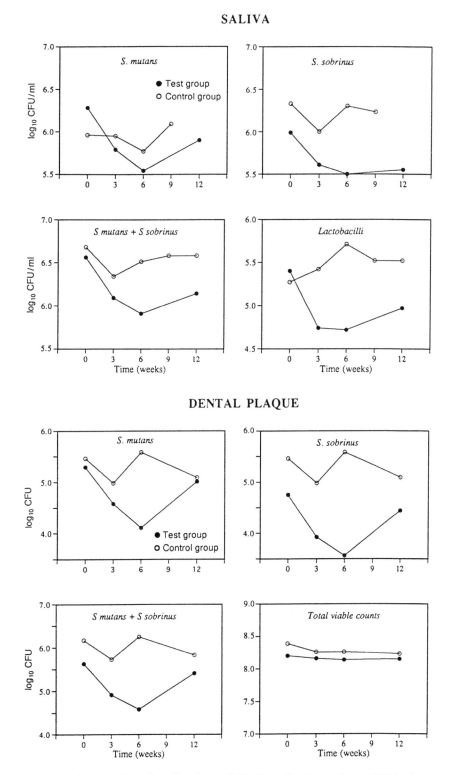

DENTAL PLAQUE

Figure 4.9 Mean number of microorganisms in saliva ($\log_{10}$ CFU/ml) and in plaque ($\log_{10}$ CFU) in the test and control groups at base-line, during the sugar restriction (from 0–6 weeks) and during the follow-up period (from 6–12 weeks). Source: Wennerholm *et al.* (1995). Reproduced with permission: S. Karger AG, Basel.

components of, fermented dairy produce such as yogurts. Two different factors in these types of foods might modulate the deleterious potential of added sugars. First, the pH of yogurt is less than 4.0, and very few oral bacteria have the ability to produce acid from sugars if the environmental pH is at this level. Second, any

acid which might be formed by the activities of dental plaque bacteria will be inconsequential as compared to the levels of microbial acids already present in the food.

The other types of food in which the presence of sugars may not be harmful in themselves, are fruit juices and particularly citrus juices. Juices

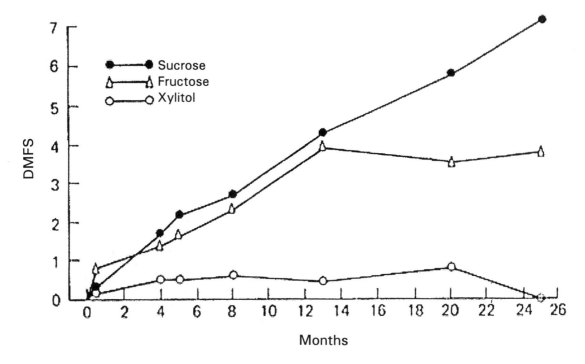

Figure 4.10 The cumulative development of decayed, missing or filled surfaces, diagnosed both clinically and radiographically. At 24 months, differences between all groups were statistically significant ($p < 0.01$). Source: Scheinen and Mäkinen (1975).

contain significant levels of sugars which potentially may be fermented by dental plaque bacteria to produce acid. However, as with low pH dairy produce, the pH of the juices will have a deleterious effect upon bacteria in dental plaque and it is unlikely that the sugars in juices, *per*

se, will have a damaging effect on dental tissues. Nonetheless, such foods, owing to their inherent low pH, may demineralise dental enamel and so be damaging to oral health if consumed in excess.

5

DENTAL CARIES: EPIDEMIOLOGY IN THE UK

5.1 INTRODUCTION

Dental caries leaves a permanent mark on an individual in the form of teeth that are either decayed, extracted on account of the disease, or filled. This forms the basis of the DMF index (decayed, missing and filled teeth, DMFT, or tooth surfaces, DMFS), which is the means used to quantify the extent and severity of caries in populations. The index can also record, at the simplest level, the prevalence of the disease in terms of the proportion of individuals in a population who have suffered the disease at some time in their lives (Downer, 1994). In the interests of obtaining valid and reproducible results, it is usual to record the index only when the disease has reached the relatively advanced stage of cavitation (caries involving dentine). As the signs of caries at this stage are irreversible and cumulative, it is important always to quote age-specific mean values. While uppercase characters (DMF) express the disease level in the permanent teeth, lowercase characters (dmf) are used when deciduous teeth are affected.

The age groups for which caries prevalence data are most often reported are 5- and 12-year-old children, and 16–24- and 35–44-year-old adults. These age groups will form the major part in this analysis.

5.2 CARIES EXPERIENCE IN CHILDREN

Much is known about the occurrence of dental caries in the child population of the UK. This comes from the 10-yearly national surveys of children's dental health conducted by the Office of Population Censuses and Surveys (OPCS), and the combined data from the district health authorities' more regular studies of caries levels in 5-, 12- and 14-year-old school children, coordinated by the British Association for the Study of Community Dentistry (BASCD). For example, in 1993, among 5-year-old children in the UK, the average number of diseased primary teeth

(mean dmft) was 2.0, but with 54% of the children free from caries, the mean number of diseased teeth in the remainder would be considerably higher. Among 14-year-old children in the UK, the mean DMFT was 2.2, with 39% free from the disease (O'Brien, 1994).

5.2.1 Time trends in caries experience in children

Caries experience has declined dramatically in the child population over the last quarter of a century. The mean dmft of 5-year-old children in England and Wales fell by over 50% between 1973 and 1983, while in 12-year-old children the mean DMFT fell by 40%. Thereafter, there was evidently little further reduction in mean dmft at 5 years of age while a very slight upswing was recorded nationally between 1991/92 and 1993 (Figure 5.1; Pitts and Palmer, 1994). In 12-year-old children the rate of decline in mean DMFT increased slightly between 1983 and 1988/89 and reached its lowest level (1.1) in 1992/93. A slightly higher mean value of 1.2 was recorded in the OPCS survey of 1993, but this small increase compared with the 1992/93 BASCD figure could be attributed to sampling error. The same could apply to the similar small increase in dmft in 5-year-old children.

Although the known decay experience of 5-year-old children has remained largely static in England and Wales since 1983 at a mean of 1.8

Table 5.1 Caries experience over 20 years among children in England and Wales recorded in successive OPCS surveys

Year	Mean dmft 5-year-olds	Mean DMFT 12-year-olds	Mean DMFT 14-year-olds
1973	4.0	4.8	7.4
1983	1.8	2.9	4.7
1993	1.8	1.2	2.0

Source: Todd and Dodd (1985), O'Brien (1994).
© Crown Copyright. Reproduced with permission: Office for National Statistics.

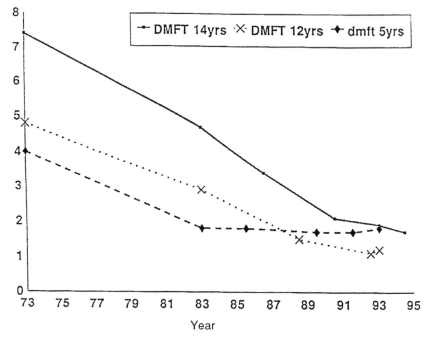

Figure 5.1 Time trends in caries experience of children in England and Wales.
Source: Pitts and Palmer (1994). Reproduced with permission: Community Dental Health.

dmft, the proportion of children affected by caries fell from 48 to 43% during the 10 years after 1983 (Table 5.1; O'Brien, 1994). This suggests that in young children, the disease is becoming concentrated in a diminishing number of children. There is evidence from a review of published reports (Downer, 1992) that these children are mostly in the poorer socioeconomic groups in sectors of the population that are becoming increasingly difficult for the dental services to reach. The same may hold for 12-year-old children. It is now clear that children from the most economically disadvantaged families carry the greatest burden of disease.

5.2.2 The influence of geography, social class and dental attendance on caries experience in children

Large variations exist in caries experience between different regions in the UK. The 12-year-old children in Northern Ireland with a mean DMFT of 3.0 had nearly three times the caries experience of their English peers with a mean of 1.2 (Table 5.2). Also, three-quarters of the 12-year-old children in Northern Ireland (76%) had caries compared with half those in England (50%).

The differences between UK children by social class, according to the Registrar General's classification, and reported dental attendance pattern are less pronounced. However, for both factors a difference in mean DMFT is apparent, with that for middle class children (1.1) being lower than

Table 5.2 Caries prevalence (%) and experience (mean DMFT) of UK 12-year-old children by region, social class and dental attendance

	% affected	mean DMFT
UK	52	1.4
England	50	1.2
Wales	53	1.5
Scotland	61	2.0
N. Ireland	76	3.0
Class I, II, III (non-manual)	48	1.1
Class III (manual)	51	1.4
Class IV, V	63	2.0
Regular attenders	48	1.2
Symptomatic attenders	63	1.9

Source: O'Brien (1994).
© Crown Copyright. Reproduced with permission: Office for National Statistics.

that of children from working class families (2.0) and that for regular dental attenders (1.2) being lower than that for those who claimed to attend only when experiencing symptoms (1.9) (Table 5.2).

Logistic multiple regression confirmed that several factors associated with social class (parent's occupation, education and dental attendance pattern) influenced the risk of caries among the child population, with the more materially deprived bearing the greater risk (O'Brien, 1994).

5.2.3   The influence of ethnicity and culture on caries experience

The 1991 Census of England and Wales estimated that the minority ethnic population was almost 2.95 million or 6% of the total population (OPCS, 1992). Approximately 56% of these were identified as being of Indian extraction, while 30% were black (Balarajan and Raleigh, 1992). Traditionally, in the dental literature, ethnic groups in the UK have been classified as White, Asian, Black or other, even though it was recognised that other important differences exist within these groups in terms of socioeconomic status, lifestyle, genetic predisposition, disease patterns and mortality levels (Bedi and Uppal, 1995). The most recent national survey of child dental health (O'Brien, 1994) did not record the ethnic background of the children in the sample, and so the only information available comes from small scale studies undertaken since 1970. They show a common pattern of a higher caries experience among the Asian than White children in the deciduous dentition, but no significant differences in those with permanent teeth (Table 5.3).

The mean dmft scores in Asian children tend to be one and a half to twice as high as those in White children (Table 5.3). It is unclear whether these differences are associated primarily with ethnicity or social deprivation; the latter in ethnic terms may be better defined by indirect variables such as ability to speak English rather than, for example, unemployment (Senior and Bhopal, 1994).

5.3   CARIES EXPERIENCE IN ADULTS

Decennial national surveys of adult dental health since 1968 (Todd and Walker, 1980; Todd and Lader, 1991) have documented the oral health of the country's adult population. For example, among 16–24-year-old dentate adults in England and Wales in 1988, the average number of teeth affected by caries was 10.4, and that mean had risen to 18.7 in the 35–44 age group. In the latter age group, 4% of the population were already wearing full dentures, so the impact of caries was even higher than the mean DMFT figure for the dentate population would reveal.

5.3.1   Time trends in caries experience in adults

The decline in dental caries among the child population is also evident among young adults. Among the 16–24-year-old dentate population

Table 5.3

Year	Site	Age (years)	Ethnic group	Mean	Reference
Deciduous dentition/dmft					
1990	Leeds	5	White	1.9	Prendergast et al.
			Asian	3.8	(1993)
			Afro-Caribbean	1.4	
1992	Bradford	3	Pakistani (UK born)	2.3	Godson and Williams (1996)
			Pakistani (Pakistani born)	1.4	
1993/94	Birmingham	8	Caucasian	1.3	White and Anderson
			Asian	2.3	(1996)
			Afro-Caribbean	1.1	
Permanent dentition/DMFT					
1989	Glasgow	10	White	1.5	Bedi et al. (1991)
			Chinese	1.2	
			Asian	1.0	
1993/94	Birmingham	8	Caucasian	0.2	White and Anderson
			Asian	0.3	(1996)
			Afro-Caribbean	0.1	

Table 5.4 Caries experience (mean DMFT) among dentate adults in England and Wales, recorded in successive OPCS surveys

Age in years	1968	1978	1988
16–24	15.5	14.4	10.4
35–44	19.4	19.2	18.7

Sources: Todd and Walker (1980), Todd and Lader (1991).
© Crown Copyright. Reproduced with permission: Office for National Statistics.

this trend seems to be accelerating, for the mean DMFT value for England and Wales reduced from 15.5 in 1968 to 14.4 in 1978 and then to 10.4 in 1988—an overall reduction of 33%. In the 35–44 age group the decline was less marked, from a mean of 19.4 to a mean of 18.7 DMFT over the same 20 years—a reduction of only 4% (Table 5.4).

An important feature of the cohort of people who were 16–24 years old in 1978 was the low increment of new caries affecting their sound, unfilled, permanent teeth over the next 10 years. This amounted to a mean of only 1.3 DMFT, and indicates the great improvement in the dental health of young adults over the past quarter century.

The proportion of the population of England and Wales having no natural teeth fell from 37% in 1968 through 29% in 1978 to only 20% in 1988. In the report of the 1988 national survey of adult dental health (Todd and Lader, 1991) it was predicted that the proportion of the UK population with no natural teeth might fall to 14% in 1998, to 10% in 2008 and remain stable at 6% in 2028. Women suffer total tooth loss more frequently than men, and the gradient in edentulousness weighs against those in the poorer social groups.

5.3.2 The influence of geography, social class and dental attendance on caries experience in adults

The geographical trend noted among children, for worsening dental health when moving from the south to the north of Britain and highest caries experience in Northern Ireland, is also clear among the adult population. It also appears that women have a higher DMFT value than men, but the social class gradient, if anything, is the reverse of the child population, with those in the more affluent classes having higher mean DMFT values. Those who claimed to go to the dentist regularly also had higher mean DMFT values (Table 5.5).

Table 5.5 Caries experience (mean DMFT) of UK adults in 1988 by region, social class, dental attendance and gender

UK	17.2
England	17.0
Wales	17.7
Scotland	19.0
N. Ireland	19.4
Male	16.8
Female	17.7
Class I, II, III (non-manual)	17.6
Class III (manual)	17.3
Class IV, V	16.6
Regular attender	18.0
Symptomatic attender	17.2

Source: Todd and Lader (1991).
© Crown Copyright. Reproduced with permission: Office for National Statistics.

5.4 THE INFLUENCE OF WATER FLUORIDATION ON CARIES EXPERIENCE

The dental caries experience of populations is related to their environment. The most striking and consistent age-specific reductions in caries levels are found in people living in areas with optimal levels of fluoride in their water supplies compared with those living in areas with negligible amounts. In the UK the optimal level, whether naturally present in the water or added artificially, is 1 mg/l (1 ppm). Unfortunately, only about 10% of the population benefit from this important public health measure. By the beginning of the 1980s, the benefits of controlled fluoridation had been confirmed in 20 countries in nearly 100 studies comparing fluoridated communities and non-fluoridated controls. The modal difference was 40–50% in the deciduous dentition and 50–60% in the permanent dentition (Naylor and Murray, 1989).

Although the general reduction in caries levels over the last quarter of a century has reduced the absolute benefit from water fluoridation, studies in the UK confirm that the relative differences still prevail (Duxbury et al., 1987; Mitropoulos et al., 1988; Carmichael et al., 1989).

The beneficial influence of water fluoridation counteracts to some extent the geographical and social disadvantages experienced by those living in more northerly regions of the country and those on low incomes. This has been clearly demonstrated by the results of the district surveys coordinated by BASCD and studies conducted in fluoridated areas in England. The districts with the lowest levels of caries among the 5- and 12-year-old children in England are Hartlepool, which has naturally fluoridated

Table 5.6 Caries experience (mean dmft) in 5-year-old children in the best and worst five districts in England in 1993/94

Best		Worst	
Bromsgrove	0.54 (F)	N. Manchester	3.96 (NF)
Solihull	0.56 (F)	Rochdale	3.73 (NF)
N. Warwick	0.65 (F)	C. Manchester	3.22 (NF)
N. Birmingham	0.71 (F)	Bumley	3.12 (NF)
S.E. Stafford	0.73 (F)	Oldham	3.09 (NF)

F = fluoridated; NF = not fluoridated.
Source: BFS (1997).

water at approximately the optimal level, and districts in the West Midlands which are artificially fluoridated (BFS, 1997). A recent study by Evans *et al.* (1996) in fluoridated Newcastle and non-fluoridated south-east Northumberland confirmed earlier findings in the same areas that fluoridation appears to reduce the influence of material deprivation on caries levels. The difference between the mean dmft values of 5-year-old children from more affluent families and those from poorer classes in non-fluoridated Northumberland was 1.2, whereas, the equivalent difference in fluoridated Newcastle was half as much at 0.6.

The five districts with the lowest prevalence of caries among 5-year-old children, are all fluoridated in contrast to the five with the highest prevalence which have negligible fluoride in their water supplies (Table 5.6).

5.4.1 Safety of fluoridation

In addition to the enormous wealth of evidence gathered over the last 50 years on the effectiveness of controlled water fluoridation in reducing dental decay, there has also been extensive investigation of the safety of the measure.

A number of authoritative bodies in the UK and the USA which have conducted reviews of the evidence, have pronounced on the absence of harm to health from the lifetime consumption of water fluoridated at the optimum level. In England, a landmark enquiry by 14 eminent health specialists was carried out by the Royal College of Physicians (1976). A total of 359 publications on all aspects of fluoridation were studied and evaluated. On the question of safety, the enquiry concluded that there was no evidence that consumption of water containing approximately 1 ppm fluoride in a temperate climate was associated with any harmful effect. The enquiry gave

specific consideration to skeletal defects, congenital malformations, cancer, allergy, and endocrine and cardiovascular disorders, and none of these was found to have any association with fluoridation. Later a working party commissioned by the erstwhile Department of Health and Social Security (1985) under the chairmanship of Professor George Knox looked specifically at the issue of cancer and in particular at the time-trend studies of two American workers, Yiamouyannis and Burk, well known for their claims that fluoridation causes cancer and for long-standing opposition to the measure. The working party concluded that the studies of Yiamouyannis and Burk were so seriously flawed that their conclusion of a linkage between increases in cancer mortality and the introduction of fluoridation was untenable. The Knox report also confirmed that there was no consistent evidence of hazard, either in terms of cancer in general, or cancer at any of a number of specific sites, from the consumption of fluoridated water.

More recently, the US National Academy of Sciences (1993) published the report of a special sub-committee on the health effects of ingested fluoride. The principal finding was that fluoride levels in the USA, which have a maximum ceiling of 4 mg/l, did not pose a risk of health problems such as cancer, kidney failure or bone disease. Moreover on the specific issue of cancer, available laboratory data did not demonstrate a carcinogenic effect of fluoride in animals, while the weight of epidemiological evidence did not support the hypothesis of an association between fluoride exposure and increased cancer risk in humans.

These, and other reports from bodies of eminent scientists, have been corroborated by several exhaustive examinations of evidence on the safety of fluoridation in courts of law. The Act of Parliament in the Republic of Ireland requiring local authorities to fluoridate public water supplies was challenged in the 1960s. Mr Justice Kenny (1963), delivering judgement in the High Court in Dublin, was of the opinion that fluoridation was safe and constituted no danger to individuals' 'bodily integrity'. This judgement was upheld by Chief Justice O'Dalaigh (1964) in the Irish Supreme Court. A similar challenge was made in the 1980s with respect to Strathclyde Regional Council's agreement to cooperate with local health boards by fluoridating the water supplies of greater Glasgow, for which it was responsible. Lord Jauncey was appointed to judge the hearings in the Edinburgh Court of Session. In giving his judgement, Lord Jauncey (1983) repelled all the petitioner's submissions about the danger of fluoridation, completely vindicating its safety and efficacy. Both these notable Irish and Scottish court cases involved the examination of numerous world authorities in the health field, who appeared as expert witnesses, and the consideration of voluminous written evidence, based on all accessible and relevant scientific research.

5.4.2   Alternatives to water fluoridation

Despite the unquestionable success of water fluoridation in the West Midlands and the North-East, no further fluoridation schemes have been agreed since the Water (Fluoridation) Act 1985. However, since that time, the whole population of France and Germany have had access to fluoridated salt. Fluoridated salt was first used in Switzerland in 1955 (Murray et al., 1991), and then in Hungary in 1965 (Toth, 1976). It is now available to populations in South America and the Caribbean in addition to Europe (Murray, 1986).

In some countries it is available only as domestic salt sold alongside non-fluoridated salt, offering complete freedom of choice. In other countries it is included in bread and may be included in restaurant and canteen food. When included in foodstuffs, it is best used at a concentration of 250 ppm fluoride, but when available only in domestic salt it is probably more suitable at levels up to 500 ppm fluoride (Bergman and Bergman, 1995). However, the fluoride concentration is best decided after careful determination of salt consumption and urinary fluoride levels in the target population. Used at optimal concentrations, it is as effective as water fluoridation in the control of caries (Marthaler, 1983).

In countries that have introduced salt fluoridation, no increase in the consumption of salt has been registered (Bergman and Bergman, 1995). Indeed, efforts to reduce salt consumption should continue, and if successful, the concentration of fluoride can be increased to compensate.

By carefully controlling distribution, fluoridated salt has been made available in both Switzerland and Spain where water fluoridation schemes also exist.

Milk has also been used as a vehicle for presenting fluoride to a population. So far this has been restricted to its inclusion in school milk offered to groups of primary school children. The concentration in school milk is usually 7.5 ppm fluoride, and evidence suggests that it may be as effective as water fluoridation (Stephen et al., 1996). Milk fluoridation also has the advantage of offering freedom of choice, but is limited to young school children, whereas water and salt fluoridation benefit all members of society.

The World Health Organisation has initiated field trials of milk fluoridation in primary schools in several countries including the UK (Stephen et al., 1996). Initial results suggest that this is a feasible and popular method of bringing the benefit of fluoride to populations of school children.

5.5   REASONS FOR THE DECLINE IN DENTAL CARIES

It is likely that there are several causes for the reduction in caries prevalence observed in the UK over the last 30 years. While the widespread use of fluoride toothpaste is acknowledged by most international authorities as a major contributing factor, particularly in those countries that do not receive the benefits of fluoridation (Bratthall et al., 1996), its pre-eminence has been questioned (Haugejorden, 1996). The principle premises upon which the influence of fluoride toothpastes have been based are that the increase in their use coincided with the caries decline, their use has reduced caries incidence in controlled clinical trials, and that alternative explanations have been difficult to find. It is recognised by many that other influences have also played a role. Although fluoride toothpaste has been the major influence in the reduction in dental caries over the last quarter of a century, it is clear that its regular use is insufficient in itself to eliminate caries as a public health issue. It would seem that, despite expensive national advertising campaigns, the sale of fluoride toothpastes is declining, and that unacceptable caries levels still exist among pre-school children; in fact they may once again be on the increase (Downer, 1994). The mean caries level in 5-year-old children in the UK in 1993 was approximately 2.0 dmft with 50% of the population affected. This situation had seen little or no change over the previous 10 years. The situation among 15-year-old adolescents was still serious with 63% affected and a mean DMFT of 2.5 (O'Brien, 1994). In a clinical trial in which adolescents were provided with fluoride toothpaste and encouraged to use it daily throughout a 30-month test period, approximately one-third of the subjects recorded an unacceptable increment of at least four carious teeth (Hawley et al., 1995).

Historical data in quantified form on some determinants of caries are difficult to obtain, while

Table 5.7 Estimates of UK population coverage by fluoridation of water and annual *per capita* consumption of fluoride toothpaste and sucrose

	1970	1980	1990
Population (million)	55.9 (*1971*)	56.3 (*1982*)	58.0 (*1992*)
% water fluoridation	7.1	8.6	9.2
Toothpaste (ml)	246 (*1972*)	380 (*1982*)	320
% fluoride	5	96	96
Sucrose (kg)	45.9 (*1972*)	37.9	35.1 (*1992*)

Adapted from Downer (1996)

on others they do not exist, so their influence can be no more than speculative. Even where appropriate data can be found, they are not strong enough or in a suitable form to permit a formal, multivariate analysis of relative risk.

Table 5.7 presents estimates of the UK population receiving fluoridated water, annual per capita consumption of toothpaste and the consumption of sucrose since 1970. With regard to sugar consumption, it has been suggested that sucrose in the diet has been supplanted by other types of sugar, and that total sugars consumption has not changed. However, information from the Ministry of Agriculture, Fisheries and Food indicates that consumption of honey and glucose syrups, for example, has remained largely constant in the UK, representing less than 15% of total sugar consumption. These time trend data are only approximate and apply to particular years within the 5-year bands reported, but nevertheless the trends are real and clearly apparent. Juxtaposed with the known mean reduction of 24% in caries experience in the 16–34-year-old population of England and Wales between 1968 and 1988, the above data suggest that the decline in dental caries in young adults is related most strongly to the use of fluoride toothpaste and, to a lesser extent, to a reduction of around a quarter in sucrose consumption between 1970 and 1990. Thus the chronological trends in the factors capable of examination happen to tie well with the data on the secular changes in caries.

Despite a considerable reduction in the prevalence of dental caries over the last quarter of a century, much of which is due to the increased use of fluoride, the disease still presents a public health problem which fluoride alone can not eradicate.

5.6 SUMMARY AND CONCLUSIONS

There is a solid body of reliable, standardised data on the prevalence and experience of dental caries in the populations of the UK documenting trends in the disease over nearly a quarter of a century.

There have been substantial reductions in caries during this period, especially among children, and the reductions are also reflected currently in lower levels of disease in young adults. Nevertheless, the prevalence of caries in the UK remains unacceptably high.

The reduction in caries has not been uniform across all sectors of the population. Levels of caries are much higher in groups suffering multiple deprivation than in the rest of the population and the differences are becoming more marked. Also caries levels are appreciably higher in the north of the country than in the south.

Analytical epidemiology indicates that caries is multifactorial in origin. Population levels are associated with a number of demographic factors linked to geographical place of residence, the environment, notably the fluoride content of the water supplies, and social factors to do with behaviour, including eating habits and oral hygiene.

Fluoride is the most important prophylactic agent against caries, and water fluoridation is the most effective public health strategy for caries prevention. Its efficacy and safety have been extensively researched and documented. However, only some 10% of the UK population receive the benefit of fluoridated water supplies. Its role in the national decline in caries has therefore been confined to residents in the fluoridated areas. Water fluoridation reduces the social class differences in caries prevalence in young children.

The decline in caries over the last quarter of a century can be attributed mainly to regular use of fluoride toothpaste although other factors are also likely to have played a part, including a reduction nationally in sucrose consumption during the relevant period.

6

DENTAL CARIES: DIET AND NUTRITION

6.1 INTRODUCTION

Being at the entrance to the alimentary system, the teeth are directly affected by the diet we consume, but also come under nutritional influences during their formation prior to eruption into the mouth. Investigations over many years have attempted to clarify the relative importance of these two issues in the aetiology of dental caries and to understand the important mechanisms involved. The overall consensus from this work is that the influences following eruption have a more profound effect on the development of caries than those operating during tooth development (Rugg-Gunn, 1993a).

6.2 INFLUENCE OF NUTRITION ON DENTAL CARIES

The evidence of the influence of nutritional factors other than fluoride, on the resistance to dental decay in industrialised countries is equivocal (Rugg-Gunn, 1993b). Before the second World War, there was considerable controversy over the role of pre-eruptive nutrition on susceptibility to caries. On the one hand, there were those who considered that it exerted a considerable effect, while on the other hand, there were those who opposed these views. Although most research workers would now agree that nutrition during tooth development plays little if any role in susceptibility to caries in industrialised countries (Winter, 1976; Burt and Ismail, 1986), some argue that it may play a role in communities that experience under-nutrition (Alvarez *et al.*, 1993), particularly affecting the deciduous dentition where delayed tooth eruption is also observed (Alvarez and Navia, 1989). Although severe malnutrition can retard the eruption of teeth, efforts to demonstrate that malnutrition during tooth development can influence subsequent levels of decay have been inconclusive.

6.2.1 Vitamin D

On the experimental observation that the teeth of dogs raised on a vitamin D deficient diet erupted with a clearly defective structure, Mellanby (Rugg-Gunn, 1993b) hypothesised that this might be a factor that increased the susceptibility of human teeth to caries. In a series of epidemiological studies, she and her coworkers claimed that young children whose deciduous teeth had an apparently healthy structure but which on more careful examination revealed a roughened surface (M-hypoplasia), had a higher caries experience than children whose teeth had a smooth surface (Mellanby and Martin, 1962). She subsequently attempted to establish this hypothesis in a clinical trial in which the diet of some children was enhanced by cod-liver oil (a rich source of vitamin D), while others were fed equivalent amounts of olive oil. Although this study, which received reasonable statistical analysis, appeared to support Mellanby's hypothesis that vitamin D increases resistance to dental caries, little further importance has been accorded to this despite a more recent study which claimed that children exposed to artificial sources of ultraviolet light during the winter months had lower caries increments (Hargreaves and Thompson, 1989).

6.2.2 Fluoride

There is a strongly held belief that the level of fluoride ingestion during tooth development influences resistance to caries, and the supporting evidence comes almost entirely from epidemiological studies. In one of the most recent of these, Groeneveld *et al.* (1990) suggested that the pre-eruptive influence of fluoride accounted for about two-thirds of the effect on dentinal caries of occlusal surfaces and about a half of dentinal caries occurring approximally. Where the fluoride content of the water supply is low, the main source would be food and drink containing appreciable quantities of the ion. However, these are limited. The main sources are tea (Rugg-Gunn *et al.*, 1987a) which is drunk by more than two-thirds of young children in the UK (Hinds and Gregory, 1995), seafood and foods containing bones (Walters *et al.*, 1983).

Guha-Chowdhury *et al.* (1996) showed that 3–4-year-old children in New Zealand consume an average of between 0.15–0.36 mg fluoride per day depending on the level in the water supply. Of course, other sources of fluoride added artificially to the diet such as fluoridated salt (Marthaler, 1983) and fluoridated milk (Stephen *et al.*, 1984), or provided as supplements to the diet (Riordan, 1993) in addition to swallowed toothpaste (Naccache *et al.*, 1992) may add materially to fluoride intake during tooth development.

However, current discussion does not involve whether there is a pre-eruptive effect, but only how important this is. The observation that some communities without fluoridation have lower levels of caries than some with, and that the probable explanation lies in the more frequent use of fluoride toothpaste in the former (Downer *et al.*, 1994), appears to support the view that the pre-eruptive effect of fluoride is unimportant. However, the explanation is more complex because children who use fluoride toothpaste from an early age undoubtedly swallow some of it, and this will become incorporated into their developing teeth.

The multifactorial aetiology of dental caries, including the strong behavioural element of sugar consumption and the use of fluoride toothpaste, coupled with the considerable length of time over which the dentition calcifies, makes an explanation of the role of systemic fluoride in the resistance to dental caries a complex consideration which is probably only of academic interest.

6.2.3 Other trace elements

Although the effect of trace elements other than fluoride in conferring resistance to dental decay has been a topic of longstanding research interest, this has never been fully elucidated. It is likely that for the vast majority of people on adequate diets, there is little impact of trace elements compared with that of fluoride (Curzon and Cutress, 1983).

Strontium can replace calcium in the apatite crystals of enamel and has thus been the subject of study as a preventative agent. Epidemiological studies have generally revealed an inverse relationship between strontium in the water supply and dental caries experience (Curzon, 1983).

Epidemiological studies point to a detrimental effect of selenium on resistance to caries, possibly by an effect on the protein matrix (Shearer, 1983). Given the interest in selenium as an antioxidant nutrient and its availability as a dietary supplement, it is interesting to speculate about a potential impact on dental health.

There is some evidence from both epidemiology and animal experiments that molybdenum has a cariostatic effect (Jenkins, 1983). Children living in an area of Somerset with high levels of molybdenum in the soil had lower caries scores than did children in other areas of Somerset (Anderson, 1969).

Several epidemiological studies have suggested that lithium is associated with lower levels of dental caries. An inverse relationship between the prevalence of dental caries and the lithium content of enamel, saliva and dental plaque was reported from studies in Papua New Guinea which supported previous observations in the USA. Lithium may have a direct effect on microbial metabolism (Eisenberg, 1983).

Although animal studies have revealed an adverse impact of magnesium deficiency on tooth development, there are no reports of an effect in man, probably because of the rarity of magnesium deficiency.

6.2.4 Calcium and phosphorus

Since enamel and dentine are composed largely of hydroxyapatite, it would seem logical that poor nutrition with respect to calcium and phosphorus would have an impact on the teeth. It is assumed that both the fetus and the suckling infant are protected against the effects of maternal dietary calcium deprivation because the calcium supply to the offspring is maintained at the expense of maternal skeletal calcium. Furthermore, serum levels of calcium are generally maintained within fine limits. However, as Waterlow (1992) has reported that small changes in plasma calcium are related to changes in growth, small changes may also influence tooth development.

Early animal research indicated that the calcium to phosphorus (Ca/P) ratio of the diet was important in determining the carbonate content of tooth enamel. The hypothesis was that a high Ca/P ratio would lead to a high carbonate content and an increased susceptibility to caries (Sobel *et al.*, 1960). This was assumed to be a pre-eruptive effect of diet.

Stanton (1969) reported a study which revealed a dramatic U-shaped curve in the relationship between caries history of 183 patients and their dietary Ca/P ratios over the observed range of 0.24–1.05. The lowest caries risk was associated with a dietary Ca/P ratio of 0.57. However, Rugg-Gunn *et al.* (1984) were unable to find any relationship between dietary Ca/P ratios (over a more limited range of 0.56–1.04) and two-year caries increments in Newcastle school children.

If nutrition during tooth development is capable of influencing the susceptibility to dental caries, then the effect in industrialised countries is so small as to elude epidemiological methodology.

6.3   INFLUENCE OF DIET ON DENTAL CARIES

6.3.1   Sugars

The evidence establishing sugars as an aetiological factor in dental caries is overwhelming. The foundation of this lies in the multiplicity of studies rather than the power of any one. The multifactorial nature of the disease coupled with the ethical and logistical problems associated with controlling human diets over considerable periods of time, negate the use of controlled clinical trials to establish a definitive cause and effect relationship.

The advent of fluoride in the prevention of caries has modified the relationship between

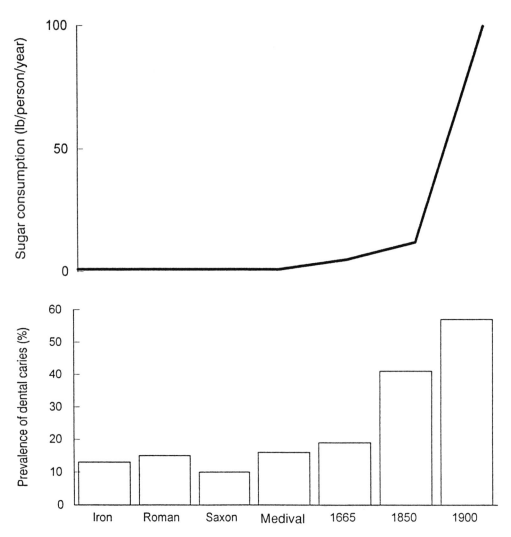

Figure 6.1   Dental caries prevalence related to the mean sugar consumption in British populations from the Iron Age to modern times.
Source: Rugg-Gunn (1993a).

sugar and caries. It is the studies in which fluoride has played little or no part, usually the earlier investigations, that have shown the relationship more clearly.

6.3.2 Sugar/caries relationships

Studies in England on the antiquity of caries have shown that historically, increases in the availability of sugar have been accompanied by increases in the level of disease (Corbett and Moore, 1976; Moore and Corbett, 1978; Figure 6.1).

Sreebny (1982) claimed that national estimates of sugar consumption could explain up to half the variance of caries experience in 12-year-old children. This suggested that for every increase in sugar of 20 g/person/day, an increase of one decayed tooth might be expected (Rugg-Gunn, 1993a).

Several communities around the world, situated as far afield as the Arctic and the Southern Atlantic ocean, have shown marked increases in the experience of caries as sugar consumption increased (Mayhall, 1975; Fisher, 1968). The deterioration in the dental health of the islanders of Tristan da Cunha form an interesting example. The islanders had exceptionally low levels of dental caries in 1937 when they were isolated from the world and lived only on locally available food. From 1940 onwards the people had access to increasingly greater quantities of imported manufactured food and this was mirrored by a considerable increase in the prevalence of caries (Figure 6.2).

Thus, in 1937 the amount of sugar consumed was 1.8 g/person/day while in 1966 this had increased to 150 g/person/day. Similar increases had taken place in the consumption of biscuits, jam, syrup, sweets, chocolate and white flour. 'The young children generally receive a poor training in dietary habits and are fed sweets, chocolates and biscuits at frequent intervals' (Fisher, 1968).

More recently, this association was again demonstrated in Nigeria where rapid changes in social structures resulted in markedly differing lifestyles (Olojugba and Lennon, 1987, 1990; Table 6.1).

Conversely, studies of groups of people with restricted sugar intake have revealed low levels of caries. The children living in a home in New South Wales (Australia) from soon after birth to 12 years of age, were fed a lacto-vegetarian diet with low levels of sugar and white flour. Their caries prevalence was 54% compared with 99% in the district's state schools (Harris, 1963). Several studies have shown that the children of dentists have low levels of caries associated, among other things, with a controlled intake of sugar (McDonald et al., 1981).

Seventeen patients suffering from hereditary fructose intolerance, who could not consume foods and drink containing sugar, had a caries prevalence of 41% and a mean DMFS of 3.3 compared with a matched control group of 14 normal people, all of whom had evidence of caries with a mean DMFS of 36.1. The mean daily sugar intake of the fructose intolerance group was 2.5 g compared with 48.2 g for the controls,

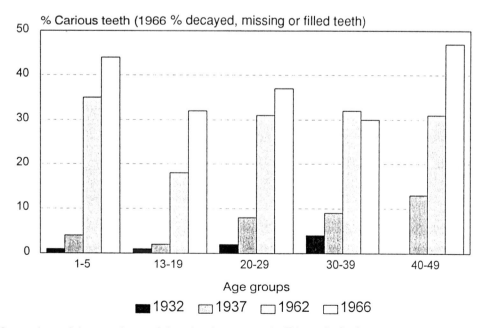

Figure 6.2 Comparison of the prevalence of dental caries among the Tristan da Cunhans.
Source: Fisher (1968).

Table 6.1 Mean number of intakes of sugar-containing foods and drinks/person/day by 5-year-old children in Ondo State, Nigeria

High social class families (urban) (dmft = 4.06)		Low social class families (rural) (dmft = 0.87)	
Table sugar	1.88	Table sugar	0.12
Peak milk (*condensed milk*)	1.20	Bananas	0.08
Africola (*cola drink*)	0.80	Fried plantain	0.04
Okin biscuit	0.74	Pineapple	0.04
Pamalat chocolate (*milk drink*)	0.68	Nicco sweet (*confectionery*)	0.04
Ribena	0.62	Paw Paw	0.04
Cream biscuit	0.50	Time cola (*cola drink*)	0.04
Fried plantain	0.48		
Nicco sweet (*confectionery*)	0.46		
Sabella drink	0.42		

Adapted from Olojugba and Lennon (1990).
Reproduced with permission: Community Dental Health.

Table 6.2 Comparison of caries levels and sucrose consumption of people with hereditary fructose intolerance (HFI) with matched controls

	HFI subjects	Control subjects
Mean DMFS	3.30	36.10
Plaque index	1.20	1.20
Mean sucrose intakes/day	0.83	4.32
Mean amount of sucrose (g/day)	2.50	48.20
Mean age (years)	29.10	26.50

Adapted from Newbrun et al. (1980).
© American Dental Association. Reprinted by permission of ADA Publishing Co., Inc.

while the average frequency of intake was 0.8 and 4.3, respectively (Newbrun et al., 1980; Table 6.2).

Populations with reduced sugar intake during war-time have shown reduced caries levels which then increased once food restrictions were lifted (Takeuchi, 1961; Marthaler, 1967; Figure 6.3).

People exposed to unusual patterns of sugar intake reveal raised levels of caries. Employees on production lines in the confectionery industry have higher caries levels (Anaise, 1980; Petersen, 1983), as do chronically sick children receiving sugar-containing paediatric medicines over prolonged periods (Roberts and Roberts, 1979). Infants using reservoir feeders containing sugary solutions for long periods also had a higher risk of decay (Holt et al., 1988).

For a number of reasons, the interpretation of the many cross-sectional studies comparing caries levels of people with reported high and low sugar intakes presents difficulties. This is due mainly to the multifactorial aetiology of the disease, and to the discrepancy between the period during which teeth are exposed to the diet and the point in time at which the diet was reported (Rugg-Gunn, 1993a). Because of this, the association between the level of caries and the intake of sugar is most clearly demonstrated in the deciduous dentition of young children where these confounding factors are minimised. Although Marques and Messer (1992) failed to establish an association between total sugar intake and the presence of caries in the primary dentition, Blinkhorn (1982) and Stecksen-Blicks and Holm (1995) showed an association between snacking and caries experience of pre-school children.

The National Diet and Nutrition Survey (Hinds and Gregory, 1995) compared dental health and diet in a cross-sectional study of 1500 pre-school children in England, Wales and Scotland. An association was reported between caries scores in the children and (1) household expenditure on chocolate and sweets; (2) frequency of consumption of sugar confectionery and carbonated drinks; and (3) high average intake of sugar confectionery and soft drinks (Table 6.3).

Longitudinal studies, where sugar intake and caries increments can be recorded in individuals, may be more revealing. In a study by Grindefjord et al. (1996), following the same children from 1–3.5 years of age, the consumption of 'candies' and sugar-containing beverages were significant risk factors for the development of caries (Figure 6.4).

Two comprehensive, longitudinal studies on adolescents in the UK and the USA found only small positive associations between sugar intake and caries (Rugg-Gunn et al., 1984; Burt et al.,

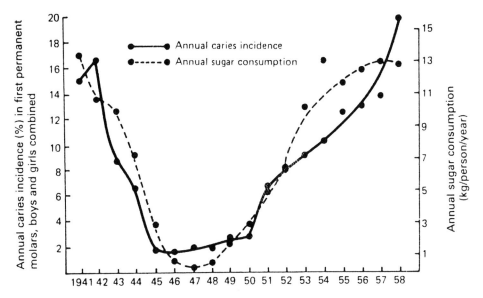

Figure 6.3   The relationship between the annual dental caries incidence in first molars and the annual sugar consumption in Japan.
Source: Murray (1990).

Table 6.3   Proportion of children aged 3.5–4.5 years with caries experience in relation to intake of confectionery and carbonated drinks

	Low (%)	High (%)
Household expenditure on confectionery	20	60
Frequency of confectionery intake	22	40
Frequency of carbonated drinks intake	25	44

Adapted from Hinds and Gregory (1995).
© Crown Copyright. Reproduced with permission: Office for National Statistics.

1988), although in the former, there was a considerable difference in caries increment between the highest and lowest sugar consumers. Both studies used total sugar intake combining both intrinsic and extrinsic sugars, possibly concealing the more important influence of the latter. In a subsequent analysis of the same data base, the British workers separated 'added' sugars from 'natural' sugars. Although they did not examine possible differences in their influence on caries increment, they found that sugar added to food and drink during preparation accounted for over two-thirds of total sugar intake supplying 15% of total energy (Rugg-Gunn et al., 1986). As over half the sugar was consumed as snacks between meals, and more than two-thirds was consumed in confectionery, table sugar and soft drinks, reductions in these foods could have a major impact on the intake of sugar (Table 6.4).

Controlled clinical trials would clearly present the strongest evidence of the effect of sugar consumption on dental caries, but for obvious reasons these are difficult to justify ethically or conduct logistically. However, a major trial of this nature was the Vipeholm Study (Gustafsson et al., 1954; Murray, 1990) conducted shortly after the second World War in an adult mental institution before more stringent ethical codes had been developed. Although complex in design and difficult to assess in detail, it did implicate sugar in the aetiology of caries. However, a limited trial by King during the same period, failed to show evidence of raised caries levels in children given a sugar intake at bedtime (Rugg-Gunn, 1993a).

A rapid, experimental caries model was developed by Von de Fehr et al. (1970), in which young adult volunteers rinsed nine times a day with 10 ml of a 50% sucrose solution while refraining from any oral hygiene. After three weeks they revealed a greater number of early carious lesions than a control group. A period of daily rinsing with a fluoride solution reversed the temporary damage inflicted.

Thus, there seems little doubt that sugar is the main dietary factor in the aetiology of dental caries. But four important questions need to be considered. First, how does fluoride influence this relationship? Second, is the total amount of sugar consumed important or has the frequency of consumption more influence? Third, are all sugars equally involved and, finally, do other dietary factors modify the influence of sugars?

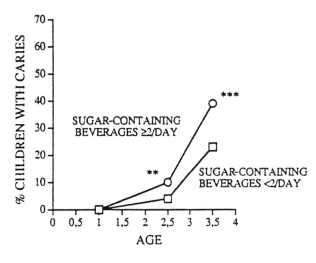
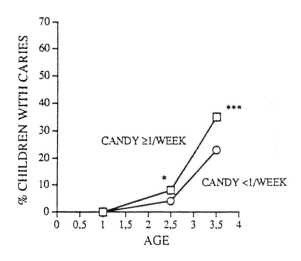

* p<0.05; ** p<0.01; *** p<0.001

Figure 6.4   Percentage of children with caries in relation to the frequency of consuming sugar-containing beverages and frequency of candy consumption at 1 year of age.
Source: Grindefjord *et al.* (1996).

Table 6.4   Mean daily intake of added sugars (g) in 405 adolescents (% in *italics*)

Confectionery	23.0 (*28*)
Table sugar	19.6 (*24*)
Soft drinks	13.6 (*17*)
Biscuits and cakes	10.1 (*12*)
Others	15.0 (*18*)
Total	81.3 (*100*)

Adapted from Rugg-Gunn *et al.* (1986).

6.3.3   The influence of fluoride on the sugar/caries relationship

The increased use of fluoride, especially in water supplies and toothpastes, has introduced a second factor in the sugar/caries relationship that masks the effect of sugar to a certain degree. Some workers have suggested that the relationship between sugar intake and caries is sigmoid-shaped rather than linear. Thus, above a certain intake, the effect is saturated causing the curve to plateau (Sheiham, 1983). If this is true then, in countries where sugar intake is well above this level, a large reduction in sugar consumption would be necessary before a reduction in caries increment would be observed (Sreebny, 1982). The increase of fluoride in the oral environment over the last 20 years has probably moved this curve to the right, increasing the safe threshold of sugar intake (Sheiham, 1991).

Woodward and Walker (1994) were able to update the earlier work of Sreebny (1982) with a more recent analysis suggesting that sugar consumption statistics now explain about one-quarter of the variation in caries experience among 12-year-old children internationally, and that this association disappears when the analysis is limited to industrialised nations where the use of fluoride is widespread. Szpunar *et al.* (1995) claimed that in a low caries, adolescent population, each additional 5 g sugar/ person/day would be associated with a 1% increase in the probability of developing caries over a three-year period.

Recent studies on diet and caries have been confounded by the fact that in most industrialised countries the use of fluoride toothpaste is widespread. Because of this, several have used more sophisticated statistical analysis in attempts to control for this. Thus, both the study by Hinds and Gregory (1995) and that of Steckson-Blicks and Holm (1995), showing associations between snacking and caries experience in pre-school children, demonstrated that this was only partially negated by the frequent use of fluoride toothpaste.

Both major longitudinal studies on diet and dental caries in adolescents in the UK and the USA used regression analysis. In the UK study (Rugg-Gunn *et al.*, 1984), there was little change in the association between sugar and caries when controlled for toothbrushing frequency. In the USA study (Burt *et al.*, 1988) the use of fluoride did not disturb the relationship between sugar and caries.

A longitudinal study by Holt (1991), in which the use of fluoride toothpaste was controlled, still showed increasing levels of caries with increasing frequency of sweetened snacks and drinks (Table 6.5).

Although the increase of fluoride in the oral

Table 6.5 Mean caries increments of young children fed increasing numbers of sweetened snacks and drinks

Number of sweetened snacks and drinks per day	Mean dmft
None	1.08
One	1.25
Two	1.25
Three	1.96
Four	1.67

Adapted from Holt (1991).

Table 6.6 Correlations between frequency and weight of intake of dietary items which are high in sugars, in children aged 11–14 years

Sweets and chocolate	0.77
Biscuits, cakes and puddings	0.71
Sugared drinks	0.86
All foods and drinks	0.32
All foods containing more than 10% sugar	0.59

Adapted from Rugg-Gunn (1993a).

environment dramatically reduces the risk of dental caries, it does not eliminate the influence of sugar entirely.

6.3.4 Frequency or amount?

There is little epidemiological evidence to throw light on the problem of whether the total amount of sugar or its frequency of consumption is the more important, as the two are highly associated in human diets and cannot be assessed as independent variables (Table 6.6; Figure 6.5).

The Vipeholm Study (Murray, 1990) showed marked increases in caries increments with frequent, between-meal intakes of sugar, but limited increments when sugar was eaten only 3–4 times a day with meals (Figure 6.6). A Medical Research Council sponsored investigation in children's homes, showed that sugar taken only with meals had little effect on caries increment (Rugg-Gunn, 1993a). The results of these two studies, both conducted during the 1940s and 1950s, strongly indicate that sugar taken infrequently with meals is less harmful than that taken frequently between meals (Rugg-Gunn, 1993a).

On the other hand, Rugg-Gunn et al. (1984) found higher correlations between caries in-

crements and total sugar intake than between caries increments and the frequency of sugar intake, while Szpunar et al. (1995) confirmed the association with the total amount of sugar consumed, but could find no association between the frequency of sugar intake and caries increment.

Nevertheless, there appears to be an association between caries levels and the frequency of sugar intake. For example, the mean caries increments of a group of young children increased as their reported daily consumption of sweetened snacks and drinks increased from none through to three (Holt, 1991; Table 6.5).

It would seem that both the total amount and the frequency of consumption of sugar are important elements in the aetiology of caries, and in normal human dietary patterns, efforts to control one will result in the control of the other.

6.3.5 The influence of different sugars

Animal and laboratory studies have suggested that different sugars may have different potentials for producing caries, with sucrose as the most damaging. However, there is little evidence on caries in humans to support this. A controlled clinical trial carried out on young adults in Turku, Finland, seemed to demonstrate that the cariogenicity of fructose was similar to that of sucrose (Scheinin, 1979; Murray, 1990).

It has been suggested that lactose is less cariogenic than other sugars, but because the main sources of lactose in human diets are milk and milk products which have caries protective properties, this is difficult to confirm in human studies involving the measurement of caries increments.

The replacement of one simple sugar by another in the human diet is unlikely to have an important effect on the risk of developing caries.

6.3.6 The influence of types of food

The Vipeholm Study (Murray, 1990), found that more retentive foods were also more cariogenic. Experimental studies measuring plaque pH also suggest that acidogenicity may be related to the time taken for a food to clear from the mouth (Pollard et al., 1996).

The presence of other foods in association with the sugar can influence the outcome. Eating cheese after a sugary food may reduce the cariogenic potential of the latter (Rugg-Gunn et al., 1975), and it is also possible that other foods consumed with sugar taken at meals may limit its effect.

Sugars contained within the cellular structure

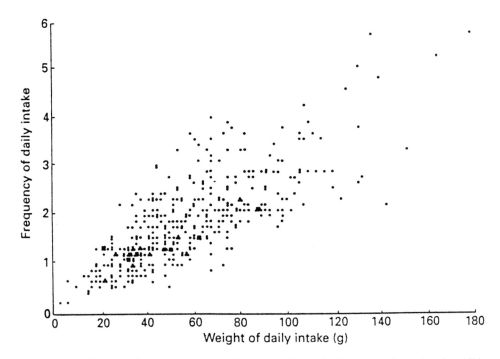

Figure 6.5 Plot of frequency of intake of confectionery per day against the weight consumed per day, by children aged 12–14 years (correlation coefficient = +0.77)
Source: Rugg-Gunn (1993a).

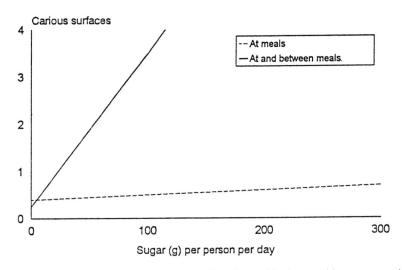

Figure 6.6 Relationships between quantity of sugar intake at meals only, and both at and between meals, and caries activity.
Source: adapted from Rugg-Gunn (1993a).

of a wide spectrum of raw foodstuffs such as fruit and vegetables (intrinsic sugars) are much less cariogenic (if at all) than sugars added to food and drinks during their preparation (extrinsic sugars) (Department of Health, 1989). These added sugars are largely responsible for the endemic nature of dental caries in industrialised and developing nations.

6.3.7 Sweeteners (sugar substitutes)

Because of the role of sugar in the aetiology of dental caries, it has been suggested that its substitution by non-cariogenic sweetening agents may be beneficial to dental health (Imfeld, 1993). Intense sweeteners are non-caloric substances added in very small quantities to food and drink in place of sugar, such as aspartame, Acesulfame K and saccharin. Other sugar substitutes are caloric carbohydrate derivatives called polyols that are poorly metabolised by oral bacteria. Although evidence suggests that these substances add little if any cariogenic challenge to the diet, few studies on humans have been conducted to support this assumption. Products that have been tested in clinical trials are the polyols sorbitol (Birkhed and Bar, 1991) and xylitol (Mäkinen, 1989); hydrogenated glucose syrup (Lycasin) (Rugg-Gunn, 1989); these all appear to be non-cariogenic, while xylitol may even inhibit caries activity (Mäkinen *et al.*, 1995).

6.3.8   Starchy foods

Most of the carbohydrate in the UK diet occurs in the form of starch in cereals and potatoes. While only a proportion of oral bacteria are capable of utilising starch for fermentation, the presence of the enzyme amylase in saliva results in some breakdown of starch, with consequent release of the cariogenic sugars maltose and glucose. In addition, the major cariogenic oral bacteria, *Streptococcus mutans*, possess enzyme systems capable of transporting saccharides derived from starch into the bacterial cell. It might be expected, therefore, that starch in food could result in a fall in pH in plaque thus contributing to the carious process.

Rat feeding studies have shown that cooked starch produces about half the level of caries produced by sucrose when fed at the same frequency (Bowen *et al.*, 1980). Mixtures of cooked starch and sucrose fed to rats have more cariogenic potential than sucrose alone (Firestone *et al.*, 1982). Laboratory studies have also indicated that starchy foods can reduce the pH of plaque (Pollard, 1996). However, epidemiological studies suggest that these results cannot be applied directly to humans.

Because a high sugar diet is usually associated in humans with the consumption of refined cereals and *vice versa*, it is difficult, using epidemiological studies, to separate the two. For example, Sreebny (1983) found a positive correlation of 0.45 between the availability of wheat and the prevalence of caries using national data from 47 countries. However, when Rugg-Gunn (1993a) carried out a partial correlation analysis on the same data, he found that, on the removal of the influence of sugar, this correlation disappeared. On the other hand, when the influence of wheat was removed, the correlation between sugar consumption and caries prevalence only re-

duced from 0.70 to 0.60. This indicates that the availability of sugar plays a much greater role in the aetiology of caries than the availability of wheat. As most cereal is consumed in a refined or semi-refined form, this suggests that starch has little important effect on the aetiology of dental caries.

This conclusion is supported by the low levels of caries reported in sufferers of hereditary fructose intolerance who have low sugar but high starch diets (Newbrun *et al.*, 1980). In a longitudinal study of the eating patterns and caries increments of adolescents, Rugg-Gunn *et al.* (1987b) showed a lack of correlation between starch consumption and caries when controlled for sugar intake. The high starch consumers ate less frequently than the high sugar consumers, however, a partial correlation analysis suggested that this was not an important influence on the results.

Although there is less epidemiological evidence on the relationship between starch and dental caries than on sugar and caries, what there is suggests that the possible role of starch is very limited in the UK.

6.3.9   Fruits and vegetables

Fruits and vegetables contain sugars and, therefore, may be considered cariogenic. However, the Committee on Medical Aspects of Food of the Department of Health (1989) (COMA), reporting on dietary sugars and human disease, distinguished between sugars that are part of the cellular structure of foods (intrinsic) and those that are outside the cell wall (extrinsic). The COMA Committee considered that intrinsic sugars are less cariogenic than extrinsic sugars. As the sugars in fresh fruits and vegetables are intrinsic in nature, they should, therefore, have little or no cariogenic potential. The dental profession has traditionally considered fresh fruit as conducive to dental health, and the apple has often been used as a symbol on dental health education material. However, the evidence to support this view is lacking.

Although various caries models have suggested that fresh fruit might be cariogenic, human epidemiological and clinical studies have failed to confirm this. In plaque pH studies, fruit juices, pulps and whole fruits containing acid have been shown to reduce the pH of plaque (Edgar *et al.*, 1975; Hussein *et al.*, 1996). The fact that fruits containing acid will damage the teeth if eaten in excess has been realised for many years, however, the main pathological outcome of this problem is erosion rather than caries (Järvinen *et al.*, 1991). Fruit has produced caries in experimental animals (Stephan, 1966; Imfeld *et al.*, 1991), but the preparation of the foods for consumption by these animals or their vigorous mastication may free intrinsic sugar from their cellular envelopes, making them extrinsic in nature.

Human studies suggest that fresh fruits and vegetables play little or no part in the carious process. Four clinical trials have failed to incriminate fresh fruit in the aetiology of dental caries. In the UK, Slack and Martin (1958) arranged for children in two homes to be given a slice of apple after every meal and every between meal snack over a period of two years. The group submitted to this regimen had less caries than a control group although the difference was not statistically significant. Reece and Swallow (1970) made portions of carrots available to school children after their mid-day meal for two years. No significant difference in mean caries scores compared with a control group was registered. Similarly, in the US, Averill and Averill (1968) arranged for young adults to eat apples after the last meal of the day for 21 months, and Bibby (1983) provided students with apples after meals for one year. Neither study found a significantly different caries increment between the test group and the controls. However, the aim of these trials was to find out whether, or not, these fibrous foods reduced caries rather than increased the disease, as it had never been considered that these foods would be cariogenic.

In two longitudinal studies of diet and caries in adolescents, both Clancy *et al.* (1977) and Rugg-Gunn *et al.* (1984) observed negative correlations between the intake of fresh fruit and caries increment (i.e., reduced caries with increased fruit intake), which in the case of the former was statistically significant.

Several cross-sectional studies have failed to correlate the intake of fresh fruit with the prevalence of caries (Rugg-Gunn, 1993a). In contrast, Grobler and Blignault (1989) claimed that workers on apple and grape farms in South Africa, who consumed large quantities of the crops, had significantly higher mean DMFT scores than workers on grain farms (Table 6.7). However, the difference rested entirely in the missing teeth component of the index and no information was given for the reasons for these extractions. It is possible that tooth erosion may have contributed to the differences observed.

The sugars in fruit juices and some of those in pulped or dried fruits must be considered extrinsic, as processing releases the intrinsic sugars. The evidence from studies of caries in humans suggests that fresh fruit and vegetables

Table 6.7 Mean DMFT scores and their components for workers on apple, grape and grain farms in South Africa

Growers	Numbers	DMFT*	MT	DFT
Apple	95	24	20	4
Grape	109	17	13	4
Grain	50	10	4	6

* All differences significant ($p < 0.05$).
Source: Grobler and Blignaut (1989).

play little or no part in the aetiology of the disease.

6.3.10 Milk and milk products

Milk is an important source of sugars in the human diet, especially for young children, the lactose content being higher in human than in cow's milk. Although prolonged 'on-demand' breast-feeding, particularly at night, has been associated with dental caries in developing countries (Matee *et al.*, 1994), studies in Britain suggest that breast-feeding is associated with low caries experience (Silver, 1987). Rugg-Gunn *et al.* (1984) could find no correlation between milk drinking and caries, but did suggest that cheese might be associated with lower caries increments.

In situ tests (Rugg-Gunn *et al.*, 1975) showed that eating cheese after a sugary food raised the pH of plaque to levels above which demineralisation might be expected to occur. This presents the question of the effect on caries of the sequence with which foods are ingested. *In situ* studies have also shown that cheese promotes the remineralisation of experimental carious lesions in the human mouth (Silva *et al.*, 1986). This action was attributed to the calcium content of cheese. Similar data for other milk-based foods provide further indirect evidence that milk derivatives may help to protect the teeth from caries. Animal experiments have also shown reduced caries levels when eating foods containing the milk protein casein (Reynolds and Black, 1987).

6.4 SUMMARY AND CONCLUSIONS

Nutritional influences, apart from fluoride intake during tooth development, play little if any part in the aetiology of dental caries in the UK. The intake of fluoride during tooth development increases the resistance to caries, but it's main influence is exerted locally at the tooth surface after eruption. The intake of trace elements other than fluoride plays little or no part in the aetiology of caries in the UK.

Epidemiological evidence from around the world establishes sugars as the most important dietary factor in the aetiology of caries. Both the amount and, perhaps more importantly, the frequency of sugar intake are associated with the occurrence of caries. Sugars consumed at mealtimes have only a limited influence on the occurrence of caries. The main dietary sugars that cause caries are those that are free, in or added to, food and drink (extrinsic sugars). The added sugar consumed in the greatest quantities is sucrose. There is no epidemiological evidence that sugars that form a constituent part of the cells in food (intrinsic sugars), such as in fresh fruits and vegetables, play a role in the aetiology of caries. However, processing these foods may release their sugars making them available to oral bacteria.

There is no epidemiological evidence that starchy foods, in the absence of sugar, play a role in the aetiology of caries. Milk, in the absence of added sugar, will not cause caries unless held in the mouth for prolonged periods. Milk products such as cheese may offer some protection from caries.

Intense sweeteners such as aspartame, Acesulfame K and saccharin, as well as polyols such as sorbitol and xylitol, can be used in place of sugar without causing caries. Xylitol may exert a protective effect.

Dental caries is a sugar-related infectious disease. Despite encouraging reductions in the prevalence of dental caries over recent years, due mainly to the increased use of fluoride, it is still endemic among the population of the UK. Its influence in terms of morbidity, suffering and total cost to the country is considerable, and a national public health initiative is required to control it. A two-pronged attack is needed before the level of the disease is reduced to an acceptable minimum throughout the country. The first of these is to use fluoride in its most effective and safe forms, and the second is to reduce the amount and particularly the frequency with which individuals consume extrinsic sugars.

7

TOOTH WEAR

7.1 INTRODUCTION

Tooth wear (tooth-tissue loss) is a normal feature of ageing, as the dental hard tissues show the effects of years of normal usage. However, a recent development has been the observation of abnormal tooth-tissue loss in young patients—the latest UK survey of children's dental health (O'Brien, 1994) reports that 24% of 5-year-old children had loss of enamel on their deciduous incisors, and 30% of 13–15-year-olds showed evidence of tooth-tissue loss. It is not known whether this development is a new phenomenon, or due to increased awareness among dentists.

The loss of tooth substance due to causes other than caries can be attributed to three processes—attrition, abrasion and erosion (Imfeld, 1996). These processes will be discussed separately, but it should be noted that tooth wear probably never results from a single cause, and all three may contribute. The term 'tooth-tissue loss' is used to avoid prejudice regarding the aetiological background to the phenomenon.

7.2 ATTRITION

The term attrition is applied to the physiological wearing away of the teeth by tooth-to-tooth contact in normal mastication or during *bruxism* (grinding of the teeth), speech, swallowing and lifting heavy weights. The wear facets occur on the *occluding* surfaces of the teeth in the opposing jaws, and also on the *approximal* surface of adjacent teeth. This form of wear is strictly age related. Deciduous teeth often show advanced attrition maybe because deciduous enamel is somewhat less highly mineralised and, thus, softer than permanent enamel, but also because bruxism is commonly observed in children.

The abrasivity of foods may accelerate attrition—this process is sometimes referred to as *demastication*. In earlier times, when flour was stone-ground (and thus gritty particles incorpor-

ated into bread), the contribution of this form of attrition often led to the near-total loss of the crowns of molar teeth.

7.3 ABRASION

This term is applied to a non-physiological mechanical process involving foreign objects. The main culprit is the over-enthusiastic use of the toothbrush, and its severity is affected by factors such as brushing technique and frequency, the make-up of the brush, and the abrasivity of the toothpaste. Abrasion may also result from misuse of toothpicks and dental floss, and from occupational factors (e.g., holding nails between the teeth, biting thread, pipe smoking).

Abrasion results in the smoothing off of the normal surface irregularities and gradual thinning of the enamel with age. If the root is exposed, the softer cementum and dentine may become abraded extensively, leading to formation of deep grooves at the neck of the teeth.

7.4 EROSION

This term denotes the loss of hard tissue by chemical etching, without bacterial involvement. The acids responsible for erosion occur in food and drinks, or arise from occupational or intrinsic sources (gastric juice). The effect of the exposure to acid, if severe and prolonged, may result in direct loss of bulk tissue; perhaps more usually, the effect is to soften the affected enamel or dentine, making it more prone to attrition and abrasion. Softened enamel may be rehardened by saliva, and it is clear that excessive oral hygiene should be avoided after exposure to potentially erosive events.

Extrinsic erosion is that due to exogenous acids—principally dietary acids (for example fruit acids, ascorbic acid, and phosphoric acid, in fresh fruits, fruit juices and soft drinks including 'sports' drinks), but also airborne acidic gases, acidic water in swimming baths, acid replacement for patients suffering from achlorhydria, and other less common conditions. Theoretically, the distribution of the erosive lesions is likely to be on the outer (*facial*) surface of the teeth in the case of acid of environmental origin, and on the inner (*lingual*) surfaces of the teeth where the acid is derived from the diet: however this distribution is not invariable.

Intrinsic erosion is caused by the regurgitation of gastric contents due to diseases such as hiatus hernia, peptic ulcer and 'gastro-oesphageal reflux disease', in which the muscular sphincter between the oesophagus and stomach is defective. In addition, reflux commonly occurs during pregnancy and in alcoholics. Perhaps most frequently, however, it is attributable to eating disorders, notably *bulimia nervosa*, in which self-induced vomiting occurs. The flow of regurgitated gastric contents over the tongue denotes the area of erosive damage—typically the occlusal surfaces of the molar teeth and the lingual surfaces of the incisors.

7.5 PREVALENCE OF TOOTH WEAR

The literature on tooth-tissue loss is confused by the lack of agreement on terminology, and often abrasion and erosion are confused. There are many references to individual case reports which relate individual forms of behaviour (e.g. dietary habits) to appearances of tooth wear, but these do not help in assessing prevalence.

An American study of 10,000 extracted teeth revealed that 18% had evidence of tooth-tissue loss, especially the incisors (Sognnaes *et al.*, 1972). In a study of archaeological material (from Roman and Anglo-Saxon burials), 30 out of 151 skulls (20%) showed evidence of extensive tooth tissue lost (Robb *et al.*, 1991). Dental hospital admissions in Boston and Los Angeles showed evidence of tooth-tissue loss on about 25%, on average, of all teeth (Xhonga and Valdmanis, 1983). In 197 randomly-sampled Swiss 26–30-year-olds (Lussi *et al.*, 1991), 7.7% had one or more teeth showing tooth-tissue loss in which dentine had been exposed on the outer (facial) surface, while 30% exhibited occlusal tissue loss involving dentine. In a parallel sample of 194 45–50-year-olds, the figures were 13.2 and 42.6%, respectively. Of the older group, 2% had loss of tooth tissue on the inner (lingual) surfaces, associated with gastric reflux. Overall, a statistically significant association was found between tooth-tissue loss and dietary intake of fruit and fruit juices.

In children, some data from the 1993 National Child Dental Health Survey have already been presented (O'Brien, 1994) (see Chapter 5). Another study showed that in a random sample of 14-year-olds, 30% had loss of tooth tissue involving exposed dentine—a rather higher proportion than the national survey in which only 2% had exposed dentine on palatal surfaces of their permanent incisors (Milosevic *et al.*, 1993). In 178 children aged 4–5 years, nearly half showed some tooth-tissue loss—most commonly, the lingual surfaces of maxillary incisors (Millward *et al.*, 1994b).

Many of these prevalence studies have used the term 'erosion' loosely, when it is clear that the aetiology in most cases is not established. The non-prejudicial term 'tooth-tissue loss' has therefore been substituted in this chapter.

7.6 AETIOLOGY OF TOOTH-TISSUE LOSS

Most of the work carried out to establish the aetiology of tooth-tissue loss has focussed on the role of acidic foods and beverages (Zero, 1996). The studies have been of various kinds: clinical trials, epidemiological surveys, case reports, experimental clinical studies, animal experiments and *in vitro* tests. Tooth-tissue loss due to gastro-oesophageal reflux has been reviewed by Scheutzel (1996).

7.6.1 Clinical trials

The administration of potentially erosive foods and drinks to experimental volunteers would not be countenanced by contemporary ethical committees, and only two studies of this kind have been identified. In 1957, a study was carried out of the effects of consumption of acidic beverages by groups of dental students on the facial surfaces of the mandibular incisors, and it was noted that microscopic changes could be identified in all groups, appearing between four and six weeks of daily consumption of the beverage. Grapefruit juice and a carbonated cola beverage caused more erosion than orange juice. Considerable variation occurred between subjects, presumably because of factors such as the manner of drinking, the salivary response and buffering power (Thomas, 1957). In a later study, the structure of exfoliated deciduous teeth of children who drank orange juice at school for 10–18 months showed slight demineralisation (Stabholz *et al.*, 1983).

7.6.2 Epidemiological studies

A Finnish study of a group of lacto-vegetarians showed that 75% had tooth-tissue loss; the most important dietary association was with the frequency of consuming vinegar and vinegar-based pickles, citrus fruits and acid berry fruits (Linkosalo and Markkonam, 1985). A further Finnish study identified the most important risk factors for erosion to be consumption of citrus fruits more than twice per day, soft drinks once per day, and vinegar or sports drinks once a week or more (Jävinen et al., 1991). Additional risk factors were persistent vomiting including eating disorders, other gastric symptoms indicative of gastro-oesophageal reflux disease and low unstimulated saliva flow rates.

Other studies have shown significant associations between the consumption of citrus fruits, apples, pears, plums, fruit juices and carbonated beverages and tooth-tissue loss. Fruit juices consumed at bedtime have been blamed for the most severe cases (Millward et al., 1994a).

7.6.3 Case reports

Anecdotal evidence has associated the loss of tooth tissue with individual feeding behaviours such as daily lemon juice consumption, or eating or sucking lemons, other fruit juices and acidic beverages. Some of the practices associated with tooth-tissue loss are abnormal—holding cola beverages in the mouth for prolonged periods, adding lemon concentrate to cola beverages, and the consumption of concentrated fruit-flavoured drinks without dilution.

7.6.4 Experimental clinical studies

Measurement of pH in the oral fluids on drinking or rinsing with acidic beverages showed a marked fall in all cases, followed by a rapid rise as the beverage was neutralised and diluted by saliva. Rinsing produced a more profound fall in pH than drinking, and grapefruit juice led to the most prolonged fall (Imfeld, 1983). In a study in which tooth sections were mounted in removable dental appliances and exposed to a cola beverage, softening of the enamel occurred after one hour. When the appliance was placed in cows milk for one hour, in the mouth for one hour, or in the mouth during the chewing of cheese for five minutes, the enamel surface was rehardened—presumably due to remineralisation of the softened surface enamel (Gedalia et al., 1991a,b).

7.6.5 Animal studies

Several studies of tissue loss in rat molar teeth, using fruit juices and carbonated beverages, have been conducted. The results are difficult to summarise as different protocols were used. However, such drinks are clearly associated with tooth-tissue loss (in this model, principally erosion), and the importance of the titratable acidity, rather than just the pH, of the drink appears to be a common theme. The differences in techniques of drinking and in the chemistry of the oral cavity between rats and man, do not support the extrapolation of these data to tissue loss in human teeth.

7.6.6 In vitro studies

Again, many experiments have been carried out on the properties of fruits, fruit juices and other acidic beverages which bear on erosion as a component of tooth-tissue loss. However, the methods, materials and conditions used have varied considerably—a factor which may have been responsible for the lack of agreement on outcomes. In general, the results implicate beverages or fruits with high titratable acidity and low pH (<4), whereas, levels of calcium, phosphate and fluoride all moderate the erosive potential. Fruit juices are more erosive than pulped fruit.

The potential effect of dietary acids as described in in vitro studies is affected, however, by other factors—notably the saliva, with its diluting, buffering and neutralising effect, its calcium and phosphate content, and its proteins which contribute to the acquired enamel pellicle. This is a 'skin' of protein which occurs on the surface of the tooth. It forms by adsorption of proteins from saliva; this process occurs within minutes after the tooth surface is exposed (for example after the teeth are 'scaled and polished' by a dentist or dental hygienist). The pellicle helps to protect the teeth from abrasion and from extrinsic or intrinsic acids. All of these modifying factors must be considered in relation to the potential erosive effects of acidic food and drinks.

8

ENAMEL DEFECTS

8.1 INTRODUCTION

The development of the dental hard tissues spans many years from early in embryonic life until the age of about 25 years. It is surprising, therefore, that nutrition seems to have relatively little impact on the teeth themselves; dental health is related more to the local effects of diet and oral hygiene than to either the previous or concurrent systemic effects of nutrients.

The nutrients which have been reported to have an impact on the development and/or subsequent resistance of dental hard tissue are those contributing to food energy intake, and protein, calcium, phosphorus, vitamin D and the trace elements fluoride, selenium, strontium, lithium and molybdenum. Local effects of foods, drinks and fluoride on the teeth are also discussed in Chapters 3 and 6.

8.2 DEVELOPMENTAL DEFECTS OF ENAMEL

There are many causes of developmental defects of the hard structures of the teeth (Pindborg, 1982), including both the enamel and the dentine. Defects in the dentine are less common and may only be detectable microscopically. Developmental defects of enamel (DDE) may be caused by hereditary factors or by environmental influences such as malnutrition, trauma, infectious disease, drugs or irradiation. This description will be confined to those enamel defects that are clinically detectable, and have as their cause some nutritional component.

Developmental defects of enamel are divided into those caused by deficiencies in maturation (i.e. hypoplasias) and those caused by disturbances in mineralisation (i.e. hypomineralisation). Their prevalence in the population is relatively high. A recent survey of child dental health in the UK (O'Brien, 1994) found that 39% of 12-year-old children had evidence of enamel defects of selected permanent teeth.

8.2.1 Indices of developmental defects of enamel

Several epidemiological indices have been used to describe developmental defects of enamel (Al-Alousi et al., 1975; Murray and Shaw, 1979), but the most widely accepted is the DDE index produced by the International Dental Federation (FDI, 1982) and simplified more recently for epidemiological use (FDI, 1992). The latter categorises three broad types of defect based on their appearance; diffuse opacities, demarcated opacities and hypoplasias. Those studies in which enamel opacities have been pooled with enamel hypoplasias confuse the issue as the two may have different aetiologies.

8.3 DENTAL FLUOROSIS

Fluorosis is a defect of enamel mineralisation and is caused by an elevated intake of fluoride during a critical period of enamel development.

Fluorosis can vary in appearance from hardly detectable fine white lines on the enamel surface, to small or large areas of opacity, and is classified amongst the so-called 'diffuse opacities'.

The condition is manifested by enamel with reduced mineral content and high porosity (Thylstrup and Fejerskov, 1978). The porous enamel is initially white but in severe cases, soon after eruption, it takes up pigmentation from foods and shows an unsightly brown mottling of the teeth. Thus, the opacities may alter in clinical appearance over time, the extent of the change depending on the degree of hypomineralisation of the enamel surface. If the hypomineralisation is extremely severe, the structure of the enamel breaks down leading to pitting of the surface of the tooth (pseudohypoplasia).

The mechanism leading to the faulty structure of fluorotic enamel involves elevated fluoride levels in the tissue fluids surrounding the developing tooth germ. During enamel maturation, the removal of protein is incomplete, perhaps because of inhibition of proteolytic enzymes responsible for solubilising the protein. Thus, the enamel crystals are prevented from growing and the enamel is correspondingly low in mineral content. The reason why the teeth are more sensitive to excess fluoride than are other tissues is unknown.

Fluorosis is more noticeable in the permanent dentition, as the development of the deciduous enamel occurs *in utero* and during early infancy; little fluoride reaches the fetus via the placenta or the infant from breast milk. From the dates of crown formation of the permanent anterior teeth, it is apparent that the period from birth to approximately six years is critical for the development of cosmetically unacceptable fluorosis.

8.3.1   Indices of fluorosis

Several indices have been used to measure the occurrence of fluorosis in communities. All of these make presumptions about the aetiology of the condition, and this has been criticised by some investigators who felt that a descriptive index was preferable (Al-Alousi *et al.*, 1975). Dean described the first as long ago as 1934, and this has been widely used in the USA since that time. There are six grades in Dean's Index but differentiating between the first three of these (normal, questionable and very mild) is difficult and open to disagreement. The index is based on the two most affected teeth in the dentition, and does not allow for the measurement of the enamel defects on the other teeth (Clarkson, 1989). Horowitz *et al.* (1984) suggested improvements to Dean's Index and proposed the Tooth Surface Index of Fluorosis (TSIF), which scores all tooth surfaces and removes the questionable category. A further index preferred by some in the UK is that proposed by Thylstrup and Fejerskov (1978) (TF Index), which has the advantage of relating the clinical appearance to the microscopic changes in the enamel that occur with increasing severity of the condition.

It is generally accepted that opacities of the diffuse type, as defined by the simplified DDE index, are related mainly to the intake of fluoride. Hence, the prevalence of diffuse opacities in the population roughly estimates the level of fluorosis (Milsom and Mitropoulos, 1990), although diffuse opacities can have other causes (Winter, 1996).

In order to detect the earliest signs of fluorosis, the enamel surface needs to be thoroughly dried, free of dental plaque and examined in a suitable light source (Fejerskov *et al.*, 1988). However, some workers have failed to do this

(Al-Alousi *et al.*, 1975) and the simplified DDE index requires that the teeth are examined wet (FDI, 1992).

Some workers have examined all the teeth, whereas, others have included only the labial surfaces of the upper incisors, sometimes adding the canines and first premolars as these more anterior teeth have the greatest impact on appearance. Enamel opacities are twice as prevalent in the permanent maxillary incisor teeth as in their equivalent in the lower arch. This is in contrast to the deciduous dentition where the maxillary and mandibular teeth may be equally affected (Murray and Shaw, 1979). Thus, scoring for mouth and tooth prevalence may vary widely.

8.3.2   Prevalence of fluorosis

The variety of indices, the conditions under which the teeth were examined and the teeth included have resulted in inconsistencies in diagnosis and, therefore, in reported prevalence and severity of fluorosis in population groups in the UK. It is difficult, therefore, to define the prevalence of fluorosis in the British population. The recent national survey of child dental health (O'Brien, 1994) recorded a prevalence of diffuse opacities of 20%. As only those defects that are cosmetically unacceptable are of public health importance, the critical time during which any factor can produce these is during the first six years of life, while the crowns of the anterior permanent teeth are forming. Unfortunately, what is 'cosmetically unacceptable' has yet to be adequately defined, and therefore measured in the UK.

Independent studies of the prevalence of fluorosis in isolated population groups with low levels of fluoride in the water supplies in the UK between 1960–1990 appear to show little or no increase in the condition (Figure 8.1).

However, there may have been a slight rise in fluorosis in areas receiving fluoridated water (Holloway and Ellwood, 1997). In the USA, where water fluoridation and the use of fluoride supplements and toothpastes are extensive, there may have been an increase in the prevalence of mild to moderate fluorosis over that period (Pendrys and Stamm, 1990).

8.3.3   Nutritional influences on fluorosis

It is generally accepted that the earliest signs of fluorosis occur at a fluoride intake of 0.04–0.07 mg/kg bodyweight (Pendrys and Stamm, 1990). In areas with low levels of fluoride in the water supplies the average intake of 3–4-year-

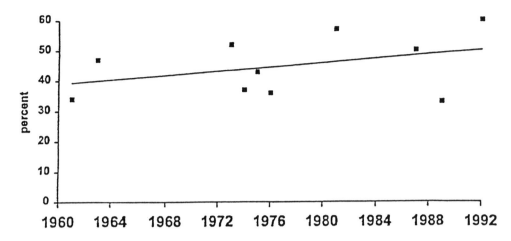

Figure 8.1 Chronological trends in the overall prevalence of enamel defects in ten low fluoride communities in the UK. Source: Holloway and Ellwood (1997). Reproduced with permission: Community Dental Health.

old children was between 0.02–0.03 mg/kg bodyweight, and in fluoridated areas it was between 0.03–0.04 mg/kg bodyweight (Guha-Chowdhury *et al.*, 1996). There appear to be only two foods commonly present in the UK diet that contain significant levels of fluoride (Murray *et al.*, 1991). The first of these is the skin and bones of fish, of which tinned sardines and salmon are the only ones that are eaten in any quantity. However, as intakes are relatively low and absorption is poor, these are not a great contributor to the diet. The other dietary supply of fluoride is tea. The concentration of fluoride ions in tea-leaves may be as high as 120–300 ppm, producing a concentration in the first infusion of tea of approximately 3 ppm; a second infusion produces less (Waters *et al.*, 1983).

8.3.4 Other factors affecting fluorosis

One of the main influences on the level of fluorosis in a population is the ambient temperature, with higher levels being associated with the increased fluid intake and reduced urinary excretion that results from higher temperatures (Figure 8.2) (Galagan, 1953).

Another important influence is the acid-base balance. Any factor causing acidosis might increase fluorosis by reducing renal clearance rates of fluoride and, therefore, increasing levels of fluoride retained in the body tissues (Angmar-Mansson and Whitford, 1990). This might explain the apparent raised levels of fluorosis in malnourished young children. Malnutrition may also increase susceptibility to fluorosis because depleted bone formation may impair the body's ability to maintain low levels of circulating fluoride (Meyers, 1978), although another explana-

tion may be that the stomach is more often empty, thereby influencing the bio-availability of the fluoride ion.

A further influence on the degree of fluorosis is the time at which the fluoride is ingested as there may be incomplete absorption on a full stomach (Ekstrand *et al.*, 1990). Fluoride taken just before sleep may also be more effectively retained, again because sleep induces a temporary acidosis.

8.4 FLUORIDE DIETARY SUPPLEMENTS

One of the main risk factors for fluorosis is the inappropriate use of dietary fluoride supplements (Holt *et al.*, 1994). Because of this, several national dental associations have revised downwards their recommendations on dosage. In the UK, a recent policy document by the British Society of Paediatric Dentistry (BSPD, 1996) has recommended a reduction in the previous regimen (Dowell and Joyston-Bechal, 1981) in order to reduce the risk of fluorosis in the critical phase of permanent central incisor development (Table 8.1).

8.5 FLUORIDE TOOTHPASTE

Evidence to link fluorosis to the use of fluoride toothpastes has not always been clear (Houwink and Wagg,1979; Milsom and Mitropoulos, 1990; Evans, 1991; Ellwood and O'Mullane, 1995). Most fluoride toothpastes sold in the UK contain 1000 ppm fluoride, so each gram dispenses 1 mgF. As young children tend to swallow about half the paste placed on the brush (Ericsson and

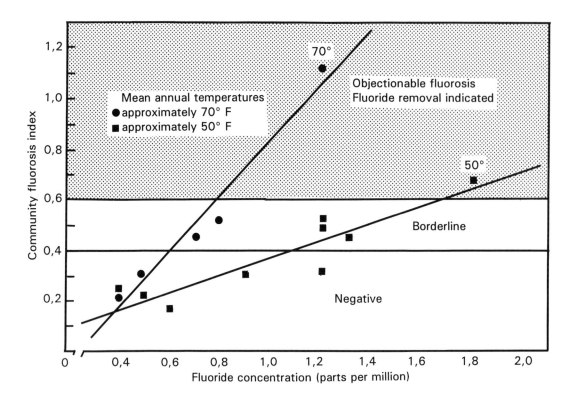

Figure 8.2 Relationship between fluoride concentration of municipal water supplies and fluorosis index for communities with differing mean annual temperatures.
Source: Murray *et al.* (1991).

Table 8.1 Recommended dietary fluoride supplementation dosage for children at risk of dental caries

Age	mgF per day*
6 months up to 3 years	0.25
3 years up to 6 years	0.50
6 years and over	1.00

* In areas with less than 0.03 ppmF in the drinking water.
Source: BSPD (1996).

Forsman, 1969; Naccache *et al.*, 1992), it is not unreasonable to suggest that this may have an effect on the level of fluorosis, particularly if they also receive an optimally fluoridated water supply (Rock, 1994; Rock and Sabieha, 1997). It would seem prudent to advise parents to supervise the use of fluoride toothpastes for their young children and to place a small pea-sized amount on the brush. However, as the effect of the toothpaste in the control of caries is related to its concentration of fluoride, a risk-benefit situation exists. Because of this the British Society of Paediatric Dentistry concluded that 'it is the abuse through ingestion rather than the use of fluoride toothpaste, which constitutes the main risk of opacities' (BSPD, 1996). They ad-

vised the use of a low fluoride toothpaste (<600 ppmF) for children under the age of 6 years who are at low risk of developing caries, and a paste containing 1000 ppm fluoride for those at higher risk.

8.6 ENAMEL HYPOPLASIA

Enamel hypoplasia (EHP) occurs in both deciduous and permanent teeth and is an area of enamel irregularity, reduced enamel thickness or even enamel absence, which is readily visible to the clinician. The area of hypoplastic enamel often becomes stained. In severe cases, much of the surface of the tooth may be affected but in the case of linear enamel hypoplasia (LEHP) a single grooved defect may be observed, most commonly in the middle third of the crown of the maxillary central incisors and the incisal third of the lateral incisors. The occurrence of defects on the equivalent, affected tooth/teeth on each side of the mouth, indicates that the defect is related to the timing of some developmental insult corresponding to the time course of tooth development. Calcification of the enamel of the deciduous incisors begins at about 15 weeks *in utero* and continues until about 4 months after birth. The most common position of the lesions described previously is usually attributed to a perinatal or neonatal insult.

8.6.1 Enamel hypoplasia in non-industrialised countries

Enamel hypoplasia in non-industrialised countries has often been related to malnutrition in children of low socioeconomic status. The prevalence of EHP of the deciduous central incisors was found to be 21% in a group of these children up to 4 years of age living in Nigeria, while there was no EHP observed in more affluent, better-fed children (Enwonwu, 1973). More than two-thirds (72%) of the children with defects had lesions indicating prenatal damage, while the remainder of the cases were indicative of an insult in the perinatal/neonatal period. A similar prevalence of LEHP (perinatal insult) was found in children aged 0–6 years in three Guatemalan villages (Infante and Gillespie, 1974). In a fourth village, the prevalence was as high as 62%. The inhabitants of all four villages were regarded as suffering moderate malnutrition, and no differences in other potential influencing factors were identified. The researchers also noted decalcified lines (no grooves) in children who were classified as having LEHP, suggesting a scale of severity of the defects (Infante and Gillespie, 1977). A high prevalence (73%) of LEHP of the deciduous teeth was also reported by Sweeney et al. (1971) in 104 Guatemalan children recovering from third-degree malnutrition. A group of 159 children who were less severely malnourished had a lower prevalence (43%) of LEHP. The insult which caused this was judged by the authors to have occurred in the neonatal period.

Children with LEHP on their anterior deciduous teeth have been shown to have a greater risk of developing caries on their deciduous molar teeth. Infante and Gillespie (1977) reported that of children 2–6 years of age with LEHP, only 31% were caries free compared with 48% of the children with no LEHP. In a study by Li et al. (1996), of 1344 rural Chinese children aged 3–5 years, the overall prevalence of EHP (all types) of the anterior deciduous teeth was 22.3%. Only 7.2% of children with EHP were caries free compared with 21% of those without EHP. Also, children who had EHP had a 2–5 times greater chance of decay in both the first and second deciduous molars. There was also a significant relationship between caries experience and low socioeconomic status and low height for weight. The authors speculate that EHP may predispose children to caries, and suggest that EHP is a predictor of caries risk. LEHP has also been associated with a higher risk

of 'nursing caries' (see Chapter 15), especially when the infant is demand-fed off the breast at night (Matee et al., 1994).

8.6.2 Enamel hypoplasia in industrialised countries

In the 1993 child dental health survey of the UK (O'Brien, 1994), only 4% of 12-year-old children were reported to have EHP. This prevalence figure is lower than that reported by Murray and Shaw (1979) in the permanent dentition of British children aged 13–14 years living in a low fluoride area. In the latter study the prevalence of EHP was higher in the permanent (8.9%) than in the deciduous dentition (4.3%).

In industrialised countries EHP, though not necessarily LEHP, has been most frequently observed in groups of low birth weight and preterm infants who may have been exposed to nutritional and other insults. In a study of low birth weight children in London, Fearne et al. (1990) found that the prevalence of EHP at 5 years of age was 71% in 110 children whose birth weight was less than 2000 g. The defects observed were described mainly as gross EHP and mainly in the incisal third of the deciduous teeth; 79% of this group were caries free. In a control group of 93 children, the prevalence of EHP was 15% but only 65% were caries free. In an evaluation of the risk factors, the authors reported that EHP was most strongly related to the need for ventilation (intubation) at birth, and was only weakly related to prematurity and birth weight. The authors speculated that the combined factors of oxygen depletion, hypocalcaemia and trauma (intubation) affected enamel maturation. The lower rate of caries in the children with EHP remained unexplained.

Preterm infants have been reported to show a prevalence of EHP ranging from 18 to 43% (Grahnen et al., 1972; Mellander et al., 1982). Johnsen et al. (1984) also reported a correlation between respiratory distress and gross EHP in a group of very low birth weight (preterm) infants on follow up at age 1–4 years. There was no correlation between EHP and gestational age, birth weight, energy intake during the first week post-partum or serum calcium levels. However, those with enamel defects had lost more weight following birth, and took longer to regain their birth weight. The authors concluded that ameloblast function may be susceptible to oxygen depletion as well as nutrient effects.

8.6.3 Causes of enamel hypoplasia

There has been much speculation about the causes of EHP and especially LEHP. A wide array of possible factors have been reported including congenital defects, infectious diseases, endocrine abnormalities, trauma and radiotherapy as well as nutritional insults at vulnerable times during tooth development, especially during the neonatal period. Protein supplements, which had been available to some of the women in the Guatemalan study of Infante and Gillespie (1974) for a number of years, were apparently ineffective in reducing the incidence of EHP. However, the authors were uncertain that the supplements were used as such, or whether they were simply a substitute for other protein foods in the usual diet.

Another perhaps more plausible explanation would appear to be hypocalcaemia. Neonatal hypocalcaemia is common, particularly in infants who are bottle fed, presumably because the bioavailability of calcium from breast milk is superior (DH, 1991) and this has been suggested as a possible cause of EHP (Mellander et al., 1982). Studies of individuals with metabolic disorders of calcium and phosphate metabolism show that only those with hypocalcaemia exhibited enamel hypoplasia, while blood phosphate levels show no relationship with enamel defects (Nikiforuk and Fraser, 1981). These authors also speculated that diarrhoeal diseases, common in undernourished populations, could also be related to hypocalcaemia. However, serum calcium is regulated within narrow limits by the actions of parathyroid hormone, calcitonin and 1,25-dihydroxy-cholecalciferol. Furthermore, serious reductions in serum calcium are not regarded as a feature of protein energy malnutrition (Waterlow, 1992), which is often associated with diarrhoeal disease. Nevertheless, a small but significant reduction in serum ionised calcium was reported in marasmic children (Nanda et al., 1984) and Waterlow (1992) stated that even slight reductions in serum calcium were related to poor growth rates.

Support for a role of vitamin D in pregnancy and its effect on serum calcium shortly after birth comes from a study in Edinburgh (Cockburn et al., 1980). They supplemented 506 pregnant women with vitamin D (10 μg/day) from the twelfth week of gestation. At 24 weeks gestation, their plasma calcium was higher than that of 633 unsupplemented women, although at delivery plasma concentrations were similar. Infants of supplemented women had a lower incidence of hypocalcaemia. At follow-up during the third year of life, children of supplemented mothers had a lower prevalence of EHP (2/30 or 7%) than did children of unsupplemented mothers (15/31 or 48%).

A logical conclusion to these studies is, there-fore, that the causes of EHP are essentially multi-factorial with perinatal oxygen depletion and factors affecting serum calcium being the most likely influencing factors.

8.6.4 Role of postnatal vitamin D status in enamel hypoplasia

The interaction of vitamin D and dental health was first reported by Mellanby in the early part of this century. She found that dogs reared on diets deficient in vitamin D showed signs of poor calcification of enamel and poor alignment of the teeth (Mellanby, 1918). Following her work on dogs, Mellanby and coworkers conducted a series of epidemiological studies on young children and reported that although their deciduous teeth had apparently healthy structure, on more careful examination some children had teeth with roughened surfaces (termed M-hypoplasia) which were more susceptible to caries. However, in a later study (Coumoulos and Mellanby, 1947) she was unable to demonstrate a clear relationship between enamel hypoplasia and susceptibility to caries.

8.7 SUMMARY AND CONCLUSIONS

Developmental defects of enamel are common in the UK, and are due to a number of factors, some of which are influenced by nutrition. One of the most common of these is fluorosis which is an opacity of the enamel resulting from inappropriately high exposure to fluoride during development of the dentition. Several indices and examination methods have been used to record fluorosis making the diagnosis inconsistent. The exact prevalence of fluorosis in the UK is thus unknown. Although cosmetically unacceptable, fluorosis has not been accurately defined in the UK. It is generally accepted that such fluorosis is infrequent in relation to the overwhelming numbers who benefit from fluoride exposure in the control of dental caries. Water fluoridated at the level of 1 ppm may result in a slight increase in the numbers of individuals with mild fluorosis, but fluoride intake from food is not implicated. There is no established evidence linking cosmetically unacceptable fluorosis to the recommended use of either fluoride toothpaste or fluoride supplements. Enamel hypoplasia is an area of enamel irregularity, reduced enamel thickness or enamel absence which is readily visible to the clinician. The prevalence of enamel hypoplasia of the permanent dentition is low (about 4%) in 12-year-old children in the UK. The exact prevalence of enamel hypoplasia of the primary dentition is not known. Enamel hypoplasia is associated with malnutrition in non-industrialised countries. In the UK and other industrialised countries, diet and nutritional status after birth play little part in enamel hypoplasia. The main risk factors for enamel hypoplasia of the deciduous dentition are perinatal insults that result in hypocalcaemia and hypoxia.

9

PERIODONTAL DISEASES

The normal tooth is supported in its socket with periodontal tissues (Figures 9.1a and 9.1b). The supporting tissues of the teeth are highly susceptible to disease, the severity of which increases with age.

9.1 CLASSIFICATION

There are several diseases of the periodontium, but the most prevalent are the chronic inflammatory diseases, gingivitis and periodontitis (chronic inflammatory periodontal disease). Gingivitis is an inflammatory condition of the gingiva, in which the gingival margins become red, swollen and liable to bleed on touching or brushing. It is present in varying degrees of severity in most of us—young and old alike—and can be controlled by effective oral hygiene procedure. The inflammatory changes are due to the presence of plaque, and in the most common form are non-specific—no individual bacterial species seems to be associated with the disease, although some organisms are undoubtedly more

prevalent. The inflammation is probably a response to general bacterial toxins and metabolic products arising from plaque.

Gingivitis may be exacerbated by the presence of *calculus* or tartar, which is mineralised plaque (Figure 9.2). Calculus is described as *supragingival* or *subgingival* according to its position relative to the gingival margin. The presence of calculus makes plaque removal difficult, hence, the need in some individuals for a periodic dental scaling to allow the tooth surfaces to be kept properly clean. Establishment of a meticulous oral hygiene regimen will, in most cases, cause gingivitis to resolve and the gingivae to resume their normal, pale and healthy appearance. Diet probably has no specific role to play in gingivitis, other than to support the development of thick plaques (patients being nourished parenterally who receive 'nil by mouth' form a thin, attenuated plaque). Fibrous foods such as apples were long held to be protective by their supposed cleansing action, but it has been found that they do not help maintain oral hygiene in

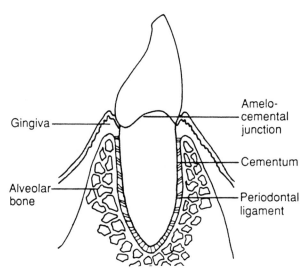

Figure 9.1a The tooth in its socket, with normal supporting (periodontal) structuring.
Source: Williams *et al*. (1992). Reproduced with permission: Oxford University Press.

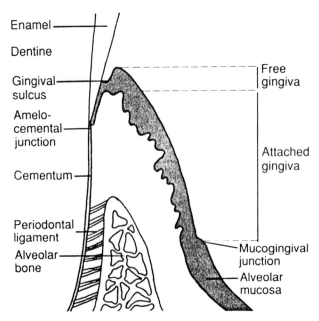

Figure 9.1b The normal periodontium.
Source: Williams *et al*. (1992). Reproduced with permission: Oxford University Press.

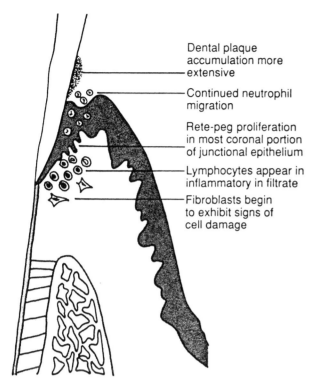

Figure 9.2 Early gingivitis.
Source: Williams *et al.* (1992). Reproduced with permission: Oxford University Press.

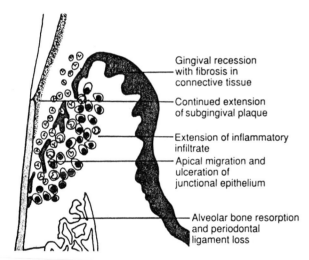

Figure 9.3 Chronic destructive periodontitis.
Source: Williams *et al.* (1992). Reproduced with permission: Oxford University Press.

the important sites at the gingival margin and between the teeth.

Chronic periodontitis is also a plaque-induced inflammatory reaction, but in this case involving the deeper structures of the periodontium (Figure 9.3). It is characterised by a breakdown of the epithelial attachment afforded by the junctional epithelium, leading to an extension of the sulcus down the root in an apical direction, which is referred to as a 'periodontal pocket'. Conditions within the pocket are ideal for certain bacteria to flourish, and there is evidence to im-

plicate these in the pathogenesis of periodontitis. The diagnosis of periodontal disease is principally by noting pocket depth using a blunt-ended, calibrated probe. Any other features, such as bleeding on probing, are also assessed in the diagnosis.

Pocket formation may extend down the root, with destruction of the periodontal ligament, and of the associated alveolar bone. The loss of attachment of the tooth may eventually lead to loss of function, and extraction of teeth because of periodontal disease is almost as significant a cause of tooth loss as is dental caries.

Pocket formation is also associated with subgingival calculus deposition, which exacerbates the effects of the subgingival plaque. The eradication of subgingival plaque and calculus is the basis of treatment, or at least stabilisation of the disease.

The destruction of the periodontium is brought about directly by proteolytic enzymes produced by the organisms involved, and by changes induced by the host response to toxins and antigens from the bacteria. Several lines of research are currently active to develop a test to reveal when active periodontal destruction is taking place—based on proteolytic activity of the bacteria, or on tissue breakdown products such as fragments of collagen or periodontal ligament proteoglycans.

Although, as noted previously, the periodontal ligament is sensitive to factors which interfere in collagen synthesis including vitamin C deficiency, dietary causes of periodontal disease do not contribute significantly to the level of disease in the population of developed societies.

Untreated gingivitis progresses rapidly to periodontitis in only a minority of patients, while in a majority the rate of progression is moderate and in some there is no progression. This indicates that there is a range of susceptibility to periodontitis, which in turn suggests that systemic factors are more important in determining the outcome than the presence of bacteria. These factors presumably include various genetic factors (e.g. variation in immune responses) but also other non-genetic factors, perhaps including nutritional status.

9.2 THE MICROFLORA ASSOCIATED WITH PERIODONTAL DISEASES

The microflora associated with gingivitis and adult chronic periodontitis has been studied extensively in both cross-sectional and longitudinal studies (Manson and Eley, 1995).

consequence of the accumulation of plaque, or is a response to specific members of the accumulated plaque. There is an elevation in the proportions of anaerobic Gram-negative bacteria, including *Prevotella intermedia* and *Fusobacterium nucleatum*, and certain Gram-positive bacteria including certain species of streptococci and *Eubacterium timidum*. Such changes in the plaque microflora may be a consequence of plaque ageing and accumulation.

Adult chronic periodontitis is characterised by the loss of attachment between the periodontal tissues and the root of the tooth resulting in pocket formation around the teeth and, often in loosening of the teeth; if untreated, this may result in the loss of teeth. For many years attempts were made to identify the specific pathogen associated with adult chronic periodonitis and bacteria, including *Porphyromonas gingivalis*, *Treponema denticola* and *P. intermedia*, were often cited as contributing to the initiation and progression of this condition. However, statistical analysis of the microflora associated with adult chronic periodontitis now indicates that the bacterial cause is non-specific. While the initiating factors are bacterial in origin, these factors may be derived from a diverse number of microbial combinations, which have specific physiological and biochemical characteristics. Adult chronic periodontitis occurs as a result of the interactions between the subgingival microflora and the host.

Juvenile periodontitis is a particular disease which affects young adults, and is quite site-specific in terms of the teeth affected. The major bacterial aetiological agent is *Actinobacillus actinomycetemcomitans* which is almost always isolated from affected sites. There is now considerable evidence for a familial tendency with this disease and for the transmission of the *A. actinomycetemcomitans* between members of the same family, and even for dog owners to acquire the organism from their pets.

9.3 INFLUENCE OF DIET

A spectacular epidemiological study was conducted by Russell (1963) in over 21,000 subjects from eight countries, in which evaluation of periodontal health was coupled with biochemical assessments of nutritional status. Multiple regression analysis of data from Lebanon and Vietnam revealed that 66% of the variance in periodontal disease was attributed to oral hygiene, 12% was due to age and only 1% was due to vitamin A deficiency as determined by serum vitamin A. The other nutrients studied, namely riboflavin, thiamin and ascorbic acid were not related to periodontal disease.

9.3.1 Antioxidant nutrients

One aspect of periodontal inflammation which has raised the possibility of a nutritional background is the putative involvement of toxic *free radicals*. These are electrically charged particles having an unpaired electron, which arise in the course of bacterial metabolism and in phagocytic killing, and are thus a feature of infective inflammatory processes. Their action is to cause peroxidation of cell membrane lipids, with disruption of membrane function; (the breakdown products of the lipids [lipofuscin] accumulate in ageing liver and heart). Free radicals are scavenged by tissue enzymes such as *catalase* and *glutathione peroxidase*, and also by antioxidant dietary components including vitamins E, C and carotenoids, while iron and copper salts have the opposite effect enhancing the chain reactions resulting in the continual production of free radicals.

The one nutrient that has been traditionally related to periodontal health is vitamin C. The vitamin is essential for the hydroxylation of proline in the synthesis of collagen, the main component of the periodontal ligament, and an important component of the alveolar bone matrix and of blood vessel walls. Thus, the oral symptoms of scurvy are swollen, bleeding gums and (as demonstrated in animal studies) osteoporosis of alveolar bone, tooth mobility and degeneration of the collagen fibres of the gingivae (Glickman, 1979). Many other animal studies confirm the essential role of vitamin C, but clearly there are few experimental studies in man. The disease state observed by James Lind, the Scottish surgeon serving in the British Navy in the 1750s, was probably exacerbated by poor oral hygiene. However, bleeding gums were observed in four subjects after 56–97 days on a vitamin C deficient diet (Hodges *et al.*, 1971). Interestingly, the edentulous fifth subject showed no gum changes, and the men who initially had gingivitis were the worst affected.

At least two studies have reported a beneficial effect of vitamin E supplementation (800 and 300 mg/day) in reducing periodontal inflammation (Goodson and Bowles, 1973; Cerna *et al.*, 1984). However, Slade *et al.* (1976) showed no relationship between serum vitamin E and periodontal disease, although serum vitamin E only reflects recent intake, and is a poor index of tissue status.

9.3.2 Folate

The gingival mucosa has a high cell turnover rate, and is thus dependent on the function of folic acid in DNA synthesis. There have been no epidemiological studies on oral health and folate status, but therapeutic trials have demonstrated the effectiveness of folic acid both systematically (2 mg twice per day) and topically (rinsing) in reducing signs of gingivitis. Vogel *et al.* (1978) showed an improvement of bleeding index and gingival index in a small group of subjects given folic acid rinses of 5 ml containing 1 mg/ml twice per day. In a group of 16 subjects who refrained from oral hygiene for 14 days, the scores for gingival exudate and bleeding index were both less severe, and both indices recovered more rapidly on the resumption of oral hygiene in those subjects given folic acid rinses (Vogel and Deasy, 1978). Gingivitis is common in pregnancy and may be related to poor folate status as de-monstrated by the beneficial effect of 5 mg folic acid mouth rinses (Pack, 1984).

9.3.3 Other B vitamins

The well documented oral symptoms of clinical B vitamin deficiencies include angular stomatitis, glossitis and sometimes mucosal inflammation. Animal studies have reported the effects on the epithelium and alveolar bone (Glickman, 1979) but, apart from the study by Waerhaug (1967), there are no reports of adverse effects on periodontal health in man.

9.3.4 Vitamin A

As with the B vitamins, while animals deprived of vitamin A suffer gingival and alveolar bone defects, there is little evidence of an effect of vitamin A deficiency in man (Waerhaug 1967; Russell, 1963).

10

ORAL CANCER

10.1 EPIDEMIOLOGY

Cancer can involve the soft or bony tissues virtually anywhere in the mouth and its adjacent structures, and the term 'oral cancer' covers various combinations of predilection sites, and different types of tumour. However, tumours of the salivary glands for example, are different in type and aetiology from those of the oral epithelium, and are usually considered separately. It appears that 'oral cancer' is usually taken to include squamous cell carcinoma of the lip (ICD* 140), tongue (ICD 141), gum (ICD 143), floor of mouth (ICD 144) and unspecified parts of the mouth (ICD 145) (Johnson and Warnakulasuriya, 1993).

The epidemiology of cancer is usually described in terms of the yearly incidence of new cases and mortality per 100,000 of a given population. Most population-based data are derived from cancer registries, established over the years in many countries and regions of the world. While internationally coordinated efforts are made continually to improve the standards and consistency of reporting (Parkin and Muir, 1992), the completeness and accuracy of cancer registration is known to vary substantially. Moreover, subgrouping of the data for factors such as ethnicity or socioeconomic status has not been extensively undertaken by registration agencies.

Despite these caveats, the evidence is overwhelming that the incidence of oral cancer varies widely between different parts of the world, and is determined to a great extent by demographic characteristics of the populations concerned and their exposure to various risk factors. Table 10.1 shows the annual number of new cases of oral cancer registered between 1983 and 1987 in a number of countries and geographical regions selected from around the world for their contrasting incidence rates (Parkin *et*

The ICD numbers refer to the World Health Organisation (WHO) classification of diseases (1997).

al., 1992). The figures are presented by gender and ethnic group as in the original tables, where specified, with the rates for gum, floor of mouth and mouth unspecified (ICD 143–145) combined. For comparability, the rates are age standardised to the world population. The high incidence in males for tongue and mouth cancer in Bas-Rhin in France and Ahmedabad in India and in Black males in Bermuda is noteworthy. In England and Wales (in common with most of Europe) and also in Miyagi, Japan it can be seen that the corresponding rates are relatively low.

Variations in oral cancer incidence, like those in Table 10.1, suggest differential population exposures to specific risk factors. For example, the exceptional rates for intra-oral cancer in Bas-Rhin (also reflected to some extent elsewhere in that country, notably Calvados), have been attributed to the high consumption of crudely distilled spirits. High incidence rates in India are associated with the habit of betel-quid chewing. The ingredients in the betel-quid (*pan*) vary, not only between nations but also communities and individuals (Table 10.2). However, the major components are the leaf of *Piper betel*, the nut of *Areca catechu*, lime, and katha, an extract of the wood of *Areca catechu* (International Association for Research on Cancer, 1985). In health terms, the key factor is whether, or not, tobacco is added to the above ingredients. An International Agency for Research on Cancer (1985) working party concluded that while there was sufficient evidence to show that the regular chewing of betel-quid containing tobacco was carcinogenic in humans, there was inadequate evidence to demonstrate that this was also true of chewing betel-quid without tobacco. Tobacco chewing among Indians carries a higher risk than smoking, possibly due to the enhanced topical action of nitrosamines, which are present in higher concentration in exudations from betel-quid than in tobacco smoke (Johnson and Warnakulasuriya, 1993). In the USA, an increased risk from the use of smokeless tobacco (snuff-dipping), after controlling for smoking

Table 10.1 Incidence rates of oral cancer per 100,000 population in selected locations (1983–1987), age standardised to the world population

Site	Lip (ICD 140)	Tongue (ICD141)	Mouth (ICD 143–145)	Lip (ICD140)	Tongue (ICD141)	Mouth (ICD 143–145)
	England & Wales			France, Bas-Rhin		
Male	0.5	1.0	1.4	0.4	10.2	13.4
Female	0.1	0.5	0.6	0.1	0.8	1.1
	India, Ahmedabad			Japan, Miyagi		
Male	0.6	14.0	6.1	0.2	1.6	0.9
Female	0.5	2.2	3.7	0.1	0.6	0.4
	USA			Bermuda		
White male	2.3	2.7	3.5	–	–	–
White female	0.2	1.2	1.8	–	–	–
Black male	0.1	3.6	4.9	0.0	16.3	12.1
Black female	0.1	1.1	1.5	0.0	1.1	1.4

Source: Parkin et al. (1992).

Table 10.2 Prevalence of betel-quid chewing habits from population studies in some Asian countries

Country	State/Region	Number	Prevalence (%)	Predominant habit	Reference
India	Ernakuluna	10,287	37	Betel quid	Murti et al. (1992)
India	Ahmedabad	57,718	47	Betel quid	Murti et al. (1992)
India	Mainpuri	35,000	30	Tobacco	Wahi (1968)
India	Pune	101,761	49	Tobacco/lime	Murti et al. (1992)
Pakistan	Karachi	10,749	15	Pan nut	Mahmood et al. (1974)
Sri Lanka	Central Province	1,133	42–54	Betel quid	Warnakulasuriya (1992)
Thailand	Northern	322	16–19	Areca nut**	Reichart et al. (1987)
Taiwan	Kaohsiung	1,299	6	Betel nut	Ko et al. (1992)
Taiwan	South Taiwan*	827	42	Betel nut	Ko et al. (1992)
China	Hunan Province	11,046	36	Areca nut**	Zhang et al. (1995)

Key:
*Aboriginal inhabitants.
**Betel nut: Fruit of areca catechu.L tree.
Source: Warnakulasuriya (1996).

habits, has been revealed in national cancer survey data. Nevertheless, snuff-dipping in the USA is far less prevalent than betel-quid chewing in India. The higher incidence rates for intra-oral cancer shown among Black compared with White males in the USA, and the singularly high rates among Black males in Bermuda (Table 10.1), are likely to be related to social deprivation which is associated with increased alcohol and tobacco use, and poor nutrition.

In Western Europe, cancer of the mouth and pharynx is the eighth most common malignancy (Parkin et al., 1993). There are approximately 2000 newly diagnosed cases in England and Wales each year with an incidence of 4.5 per 100,000 (Office of Population Censuses and Surveys, 1994). In the UK, it represents 1–2% of total cancer incidence. Although oral cancer is a relatively small health care problem, morbidity and mortality from the disease are high, with

(ICD 141, 143-146.)

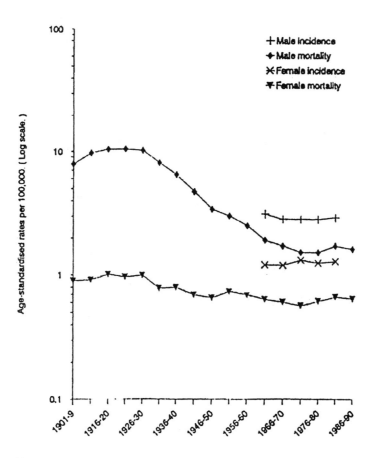

Figure 10.1 Oral cancer 1901–1990.
Source: Hindle *et al.* (1996). Reproduced with permission: Brit J Oral Maxillofacial Surg.

over 60% of patients dying as a result of their oral lesions (Platz *et al.*, 1986). There is also evidence that oral cancer is increasing in the UK (Hindle *et al.*, 1996; Macfarlane *et al.*, 1992), elsewhere in Europe, and in Australia (Macfarlane, 1993). Figures 10.1–10.4 graphically illustrate the changes in oral cancer incidence and mortality in England and Wales during the present century (Hindle *et al.*, 1996). Figure 10.1 considers males and females separately, while Figure 10.2 depicts the incidence and mortality data for males only, divided into the 35–64 and 65+ years age groups. The mortality and incidence for males, displayed by birth cohort in Figures 10.3 and 10.4, respectively, support the suggestion of an increase in oral cancer in those under 60 years of age in the birth periods shown.

Oral cancer incidence increases with age. The rates for carcinoma of the gum, floor of the mouth and unspecified parts of the mouth among males in England and Wales, for ex-

ample, rises steadily from 0.1 per 100,000 in the 25–29 years age group to 12.3 per 100,000 in those aged 85 years or over (Parkin *et al.*, 1992). Males in a given population almost invariably have higher age-specific incidence rates than females for all types of predilection site. In England and Wales, the tongue (usually the lateral border) is the most frequently involved oral site, while the floor of the mouth ranks second with about half the number of cases (Johnson and Warnakulasuriya, 1993). Other sites at risk are the lower buccal sulcus, alveolus and angle of the mouth (Speight and Morgan, 1993).

10.2 BETEL-QUID AND TOBACCO CHEWING AMONG THE UK'S MINORITY ETHNIC COMMUNITY

Betel-quid chewing is widespread in the Indian subcontinent but only a small amount of data

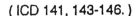

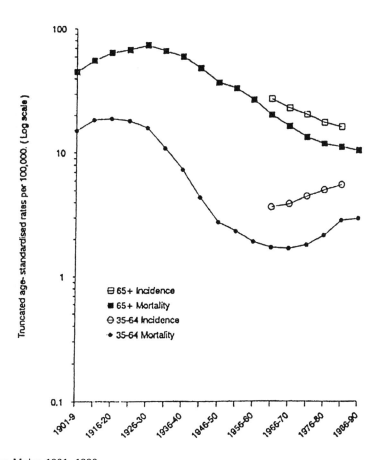

Figure 10.2 Oral cancer. Males 1901–1990.
Source: Hindle *et al.* (1996). Reproduced with permission: Brit J Oral Maxillofacial Surg.

exists about this behaviour among the Asian ethnic community resident in the UK (Table 10.3). For a number of years, there has been the belief among health workers that the inclusion of tobacco into the betel-quid occurs primarily among the Bangladeshi community. This observation has been confirmed in the recent Health Education Report 'Black and Minority Ethnic Groups in England' (Health Education Authority, 1994; Table 10.4).

The high levels of recorded betel-quid and tobacco chewing among the Bangladeshi community has not led to detailed systematic research on the extent of oral cancer and precancerous lesions among this population. This is despite clear evidence from the medical literature that populations in India suffer higher rates of this condition than other groups. There is, however, evidence emerging that the UK's South Asian community do have a higher risk of oral cancer mortality. Swerdlow *et al.* (1995)

explored the risk of cancer mortality from 1973–1985 in persons born in the Indian subcontinent who migrated to England and Wales (Indian ethnic immigrants), and compared this with cancer mortality of British-born Indians, using data from England and Wales death certificates. There were substantive and highly significant increased risks in Indian immigrants for cancers of the mouth and pharynx, gall bladder and liver in each sex; larynx and thyroid in males and oesophagus in females. The authors concluded that the results suggest the need for public health measures to combat the high risks of oral and pharyngeal cancers in the Indian immigrant population by the prevention of betel-quid chewing. The statutory recording of ethnic background in cancer registers began in April 1995 and exploration of this information will highlight whether, or not, oral cancer rates are higher among the UK's ethnic minority population.

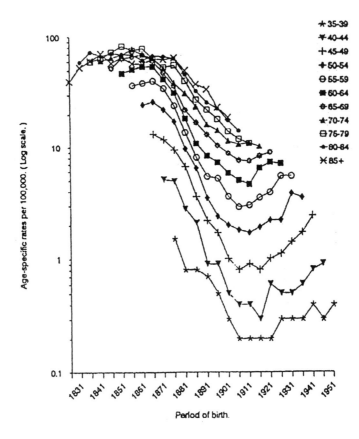

Figure 10.3 Oral cancer mortality. Males. (Birth Cohorts 1827–1951).
Source: Hindle *et al.* (1996). Reproduced with permission: Brit J Oral Maxillofacial Surg.

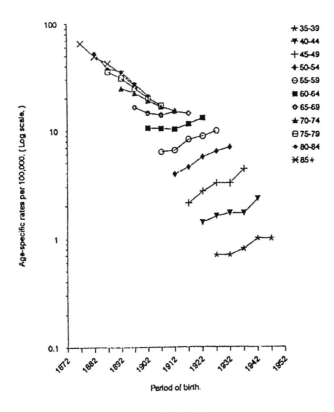

Figure 10.4 Oral cancer incidence. Males. (Birth Cohorts 1877–1947).
Source: Hindle *et al.* (1996). Reproduced with permission: Brit J Oral Maxillofacial Surg.

Table 10.3 Prevalence of betel-quid chewing habit in ethnic minority groups in the UK

Region	Number	Community	Habit	Prevalence (%)	Reference
West Yorkshire	296	Bangladeshi	Pan	95	Summers et al. (1994)
			Zarda	27	
Birmingham	334	Bangladeshi	Betel-quid	92–96	Bedi and Gilthorpe (1995)
Inner London	158	Bangladeshi	Betel-quid	78	Pearson (1994)
Outer London	183	Mixed Asian*	Betel-quid	47	Atwal (1995)

* Predominant Indian.
Source: Warnakulasuriya (1996).

Table 10.4 Chewing tobacco products by gender and age group

			Women			Men		
		All %	16–29%	30–49%	50–74%	16–29%	30–49%	50–74%
Any chewing	Indian	15	6	12	17	10	23	23
product	Pakistani	7	7	10	8	4	7	11
	Bangladeshi	66	43	88	96	49	76	74
Paan	Indian	10	5	8	11	8	16	16
	Pakistani	4	5	6	1	2	5	5
	Bangladeshi	50	31	59	76	40	58	62
Any tobacco	Indian	4	2	3	4	1	3	12
product	Pakistani	1	1	1	2	1	1	2
	Bangladeshi	28	14	48	58	13	31	31
Betel nut/	Indian	3	<0.5	3	4	1	3	8
sopari chewed	Pakistani	<0.5	1	0	0	0	<0.5	0
with tobacco	Bangladeshi	27	13	48	58	12	29	31
Betel nut/	Indian	4	2	4	1	2	5	7
sopari	Pakistani	1	3	3	0	0	1	0
chewed with	Bangladeshi	35	28	39	36	24	47	43
no tobacco								

Source: Health Education Authority (1994). Reproduced with permission.

10.3 CLINICAL FEATURES OF ORAL CANCER

10.3.1 Squamous cell carcinoma

Clinically, oral carinomas may be exophytic, but most present as persistent ulcers. Ninety percent of intra-oral carcinomas arise on the lateral border of the tongue or the floor of the mouth, and persistent lesions should be biopsied where clinical doubt exists. Early diagnosis is particularly important, since excision of small lesions is usually curative. Oral carcinomas metastasise in the first instance to regional lymph nodes. Haematogenous spread is an uncommon early event. Treatment of larger lesions is by surgical excision and/or radiotherapy, and less com-monly chemotherapy. The prognosis for larger lesions is poor.

10.3.2 Oral precancer

Although oral cancer often apparently arises *de novo*, there are a number of clinically identifiable precursor lesions which constitute a detectable preclinical phase in about 10% of cases. The most important of these are leukoplakia, erythro-plakia and lichen planus. Leukoplakia is defined by the WHO as a white patch of oral mucosa which cannot be scraped off (thus excluding, for example, pseudomembranous candidiasis), and cannot be attributed to any other cause. Poten-tially malignant lesions, such as leukoplakia and other conditions associated with a high risk, may be present in up to 5% of the population over 40 years of age in industrialised countries (Axéll, 1987; Bánóczy and Rigo, 1991; Bouquot and Gorlin, 1986; Kleinman *et al.*, 1991). However, their rates of malignant transformation are generally low. The proportion of leukoplakias, which have been reported as undergoing malignant change in follow-up studies, varies from 0.1 to about 10% (Einhorn and Wersäll, 1967; Bánóczy, 1977; Silverman *et al.*, 1976). An overall rate of transformation of 2–4% for leukoplakia and 1% for lichen planus could be regarded as reasonable estimates for industrialised countries. It has also been established that a patient with leukoplakia has a greater chance of developing cancer than a person without a lesion, with an estimated relative risk of seven in women and around five in men (Silverman *et al.*, 1976). In addition, about 3–6% of patients have lesions clinically diagnosed as leukoplakia, which are found at biopsy to be carcinoma (Waldron and Shafer, 1975).

It may take 10–15 years for a leukoplakia to progress to oral cancer (Speight and Morgan, 1993), although it is impossible to accurately predict from their clinical appearance those lesions that will progress. Leukoplakia lesions show a variable degree of epithelial dysplasia on histological examination, although in contrast to neoplasia of the uterine cervix, there is no evidence of regular progression through severe dysplasia to frank carcinoma. In addition, there is no evidence to support a viral aetiology for oral carcinoma. The most important determinant of the relative risk of malignant change is the presence of epithelial dysplasia on histological examination; various clinical features of leukoplakia to do with colour (red speckling), texture (roughened, nodular surface) and the presence of erythematous areas (erythroplakia), correlate to some extent with degrees of severity of dysplastic change. The location of lesions is also significant. The lateral border of the tongue, floor of the mouth, lower buccal sulcus and alveolus, and the angle of the mouth are the sites most at risk (Speight and Morgan, 1993). The sites where lichen planus is most at risk of progressing to malignancy are also the tongue and gingiva. Because of the potentially lethal nature of precancerous lesions, which are generally without symptoms of pain or discomfort, it is important that apparently healthy people with the disease are identified and kept under continuing clinical supervision. Careful follow-up of premalignant lesions is mandatory.

10.4   FACTORS RELATED TO ORAL CANCER

Causative or aetiological agents for cancer are those for which laboratory or epidemiological evidence is available to support a carcinogenic potential. Elements of the diet and nutritional deficiencies are among known lifestyle-related determinants of oral cancer and risk factors for the disease. La Vecchia *et al.* (1993) take the view that one in six oral cancers in Europe are due to dietary deficiencies or imbalances, while Macfarlane (1993), in an extensive review of the literature, concluded that the combined effects of tobacco smoking and alcohol consumption, moderated by the protection afforded from intakes of fruit and vegetables, appear to explain the great majority of oral cancer cases in Europe, the USA and Australasia.

10.5   LIMITATIONS OF TIME SERIES DATA

Examination of time-series data relating historical changes in supposed determinants and risk factors to trends in disease incidence and mortality, is a well established method for the epidemiological investigation of the aetiology of cancer. However, the utility of statistics on population consumption of various dietary elements and micronutrients in analytical epidemiology, is limited. It is not possible to relate changes in population consumption to changes in the consumption pattern of individuals. Moreover, aggregated population data do not allow separate analyses by gender, age group, socioeconomic classification or geographical subset, whereas, it is known that consumption of alcohol, for example, is likely to vary greatly between such demographic strata. Nevertheless, in the absence of alternative sources of information, time-series analysis can provide useful insight into the association between the incidence of oral cancer, and previous consumption patterns and exposures in respect of factors which affect the occurrence of the disease. It is the basis of some of the most powerful studies cited in the following sections.

10.6   ALCOHOL AND TOBACCO

In Western society and elsewhere, the recreational use of alcohol is often associated with the habit of tobacco smoking. In investigating the aetiology of oral cancer in relation to dietary factors, it is important to separate and isolate the possible independent effects of each of these risk factors, as well as considering their combined impact.

The precise role of alcohol remains to be established (Smith, 1989; Van Wyk, 1982) but, like tobacco, it has been consistently found to be an important independent risk factor for intra-oral tumours, and also hypopharyngeal and oropharyngeal cancer (Blot et al., 1988; Brugere et al., 1986; Graham et al., 1977; Keller and Terris, 1965; Merletti et al., 1989; Tuyns et al., 1988; Wynder et al., 1957; Young et al., 1986). An interaction between alcohol and tobacco has also been reported, with evidence that their combined effect is greater than the sum of the risks from exposure to either on its own (Brugere et al., 1986; Franceschi et al., 1990; Rothman and Keller, 1972). Elwood et al. (1984) found the association between alcohol and oral cancer to be strong, highly significant and more important than smoking.

However, attempting to establish the magnitude of the relative risks of oral cancer from tobacco smoking and alcohol consumption using data from published case-control studies is no easy task. The findings are sometimes inconsistent or even conflicting. The difficulties arise from a number of sources. These include variable sample sizes, which oral sites are included, methods of measuring consumption, and the units of consumption used. Again, while most studies control for age and gender, there is a variation in the other confounding factors that are, or are not, controlled in the regression analyses. Table 10.5 presents selected findings from a number of relevant studies in order to elucidate the nature of the relationships between tobacco smoking, alcohol drinking and oral cancer. These are illustrated diagrammatically in Figure 10.5 (Cancer Research Campaign, 1993).

There has been no consistent difference reported between the magnitude of the effect of the two main risk factors for carcinoma of the hypopharynx and oropharynx, and the adjacent sites of tongue and mouth. Tobacco and alcohol appear to be the shared common risk factors (Macfarlane, 1993). Among intra-oral sites, tobacco has been demonstrated as being associated more with soft-palate lesions, while alcohol is associated with lesions of the floor of the mouth and tongue (Boffeta et al., 1992).

10.6.1 Types of alcoholic beverage

Consideration has been given to the relative malignant potential of the various types of alcoholic beverage. In a case-control study of patients with histologically confirmed oral dysplasia, there was some indication that spirits might be more closely associated with dysplastic lesions than other types of alcoholic drink (Kulasegaram et al., 1995). Blot et al. (1988), Macfarlane (1993) and Merletti et al. (1989) produced evidence that spirits and beer were more important risk factors for oral cancer than wine, although other workers have found the highest risks to be associated with wine consumption (Franco et al., 1989; Barra et al., 1990). Barra and coworkers concluded that it is the most frequently consumed beverage in any area that appears mostly to increase risk. Apparent variations in risk according to the type of alcoholic drink may be due to the ethanol content and differing impurities, including nitrosamines, many of which are carcinogenic (Johnson and Warnakulasuriya, 1993). Mashberg et al. (1993) and Doll (1992) take the view that there is no difference in risk potential between different types of alcoholic beverage. Available UK national data for the consumption of alcohol show that an increase has occurred for beer, for wine and for spirits since around 1960 (Spring and Buss, 1977).

10.6.2 Dose-risk relationship

Several studies, previously cited, demonstrate that the risk of oral cancer increases according to the amount of alcohol consumed (Keller and Terris, 1965; Rothman and Keller, 1972; Wynder et al., 1957). More recent, large case-control studies, with the ability to control for confounding factors, have affirmed a dose-risk relationship (Barra et al., 1990; Blot et al., 1988; Franco et al., 1989; Merletti et al., 1989). Increased mortality from oral and pharyngeal cancer has been observed in occupations associated with a high alcohol intake and, in a number of countries, alcoholics have been found to have a high relative risk of oral cancer compared to the general population (Monson and Lyon, 1975; Schmidt and Popham, 1981; Sundby, 1967). Prospective studies have shown that individuals with the highest alcohol consumption levels have an increased incidence of, and mortality from, the disease relative to abstainers (Kato et al., 1992; Klatsky et al., 1981).

10.6.3 Trends in alcohol consumption

Macfarlane (1993) has undertaken a detailed review of time trends in alcohol consumption in the UK and three other countries (Slovakia, Sweden and Australia) where registration data show an increase in oral cancer incidence. His findings throw some important light on the role

Table 10.5 Summary of investigations of the relationships between tobacco smoking, alcohol drinking and oral cancer

Sites included (ICD codes)	Cases No. controls No. M and/or F	Variables controlled	Tobacco intake	Alcohol intake	Tobacco + alcohol − RR or OR	Tobacco − alcohol + RR or OR	Tobacco + alcohol + RR or OR	Reference
Incidence: 141, 143–146, 148, 149	732 M / 837 M	Race, age, location	Non-smoker vs 40+/day for 20+ year	<1 drink/week vs 30+ drink/week	7.4	5.8	37.7	Blot et al. (1988)
Incidence: 141, 143–145	352 M + F / 464 M + F	Age, gender, location	<1 pack-years vs >1000 pack-years	<1 kg lifetime vs >100 kg lifetime	15.2	23.1	141.6	Franco et al. (1989)
Incidence: 140, 141, 143–145	584 M / 1222 M	Adequacy of dentition	Never vs >1 pack/day	<14 drinks/week vs ≥14 drinks/week	1.54	1.70	2.49	Graham et al. (1977)
Histologically confirmed oral dysplasia	70 M + F / 70 M + F	Age, gender ethnicity	Non-smoker vs 20+ cigs/day	Non-drinker vs drinker	13.5	0.65	–	Kulasegaram et al. (1995)
Incidence: 141, 144, 146	290 M + F / 290 M + F	Age, gender, social class	Non-smoker vs 51–70 pack-years	Lowest quintile vs highest quintile	7.7	14.8	–	Marshall et al. (1992)
Incidence: oral cavity, oropharynx	359 M / 2280 M	Age	≤5 cigs/day vs 36+ cigs/day	≤1 WE/day* vs 11–21 WE/day	3.2	12.5	98.4	Mashberg et al. (1993)
Incidence: 140, 141, 143–146	86 M / 385 M	Age	<8 g/day vs >16 g/day	<41 g/day vs ≥41 g/day	2.5	0.6	21.4	Merletti et al. (1989)
Incidence: mouth, pharynx	483 M / 477 M	Age, gender	Non-smoker vs 40+ cigs/day	Non-drinker vs 1.6+ oz/day	2.43	2.33	15.5	Rothman and Keller (1972)
Incidence: lip, mouth, pharynx	543 M / 543 M	Age, gender, education	<16 cigs/day vs 34+ cigs/day	<1 unit/day vs >6 unit/day	8.40	9.69	19.4	Wynder et al. (1957) (modified by Rothman and Keller, 1972)

Key:
* WE = whiskey equivalent = 1 oz (29.57 ml) of 86-proof hard liquor (10.24 g alcohol).
RR = relative risk.
OR = odds ratio.
M = male, F = female.

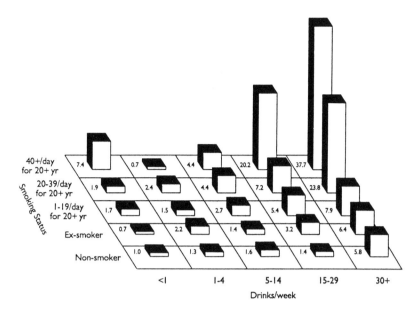

Figure 10.5 Relative risk of oral/pharyngeal cancer in males by alcohol and tobacco consumption.
Source: Cancer Research Campaign (1993).

of alcohol in relation to the occurrence of the disease. Quoting data from Spring and Buss (1977), he states that ethanol consumption per head of the UK population was estimated to have fallen from around 25 g per person per day throughout the nineteenth century, to a low of about 10 g between 1930 and 1960. However, data from the International Agency for Research on Cancer (1988) showed that the average consumption of ethanol in the UK increased by about 40% between 1960 and 1985. Macfarlane concluded that it was likely that part of the increased incidence of intra-oral cancer was due to this rise in alcohol consumption.

Summarising the remainder of the findings, alcohol consumption has risen substantially in Slovakia during the past 40 years. Increases in beer intake occurred up to about 1965, when consumption levels were estimated to be 106 litres per head annually compared with 53.7 litres in 1953. A large increase in spirit consumption was confined primarily to the period between 1964 (3.7 litres per head) and 1977 (11.0 litres per head) with little change thereafter. Large increases in alcohol consumption have also occurred in Sweden. Between the mid-1930s and 1980, annual wine consumption increased ten-fold to 9.5 litres per adult. Beer intakes doubled to 48.6 litres and spirits increased from 4.5 to 5.6 litres. In Australia, there was a three-fold increase in total ethanol consumption between 1930 and the early 1980s, after which a decrease of about 10% occurred. In all three countries, as in the UK, registration data show that oral cancer incidence has increased since the 1960s, particularly in adults under 60 years of age.

In addition to the above countries, Møller (1989) reported a rise in oral cancer in Denmark for those born after 1908 and ascribed this to increasing alcohol consumption rather than tobacco consumption. Similar comments have been made in relation to England and Wales (Hindle *et al.*, 1996; Hindle and Nally, 1991) and Scotland (Macfarlane *et al.*, 1992).

10.7 DIETARY FACTORS

Apart from the important risk associated with high alcohol consumption, several constituents of the diet have been implicated in the aetiology of oral cancer, while others may have a role in its prevention. The most common findings are of decreased risks with an increasing intake of fresh fruit and yellow-green vegetables (Winn *et al.*, 1984; McLaughlin *et al.*, 1988). Recent shifts towards diets containing a higher proportion of these items, among some sections of the population at least, may result in a lowering as opposed to a heightening of risk.

10.7.1 Iron deficiency

A disorder, known in the UK as the Kelly-Paterson syndrome (also the Plummer-Vinson syndrome), is related to iron deficiency anaemia. The condition is characterised by thinning and atrophy of the mucosal lining of the upper gastro-intestinal tract, with accompanying dysphagia. It is associated with malignancies in the upper alimentary tract, and epidemiological studies have shown that there is also an increased risk of oral and pharyngeal cancers

(Smith, 1973; Larsson *et al.*, 1975; Wynder and Fryer, 1958). Middle-aged women are particularly prone to this condition. In Sweden, it has been noted that a fall in the incidence of sideropenic anaemia coincided with a fall in the incidence of oral and pharyngeal carcinoma (Larsson *et al.*, 1975). Elsewhere, elderly women with intra-oral cancer, who claimed never to have used tobacco or alcohol, were shown to have significantly lower serum iron levels than control subjects (Rich and Radden, 1984). There is a higher susceptibility to oral cancer in deficiency states (Warnakulasuriya and Prabhu, 1992), and it is possible that riboflavin, thiamin, pyridoxine and protein deficiencies are also associated with the Kelly-Paterson syndrome.

10.7.2 Vitamins

A relationship suggesting a protective effect against oral cancer has been demonstrated for various vitamins, notably A, B-group, C and E (McLaughlin *et al.*, 1988; Zheng *et al.*, 1993), and β-carotene (La Vecchia *et al.*, 1991), with the strongest protection appearing to be afforded by fresh fruit (McLaughlin *et al.*, 1988). Unfortunately, as already discussed, the problem of assessing dietary intake of vitamins in individual subjects is difficult, particularly when attempting to evaluate past dietary patterns, so that the validity of research in this area depends to a large extent on the accuracy of self-reporting of behaviour. It is also necessary to control for the confounding effects of alcohol and tobacco use.

Geographically, there is some suggestion of an inverse relationship between fresh fruit consumption and the incidence of intra-oral cancer in males in different regions of England (Hindle, personal communication). In women, Braddon *et al.* (1988) showed that the average daily vitamin C intake is significantly lower in Wales and the north of England than in southeast England, although data from East Anglia were conflicting. No firm conclusions can be drawn, but it appears that regional variations in the dietary intake of some micronutrients may be implicated in the geographic distribution of intra-oral cancer in England and Wales.

The observations regarding certain micronutrients, including vitamin A and analogues (isotretinoin, for example), suggested that these might have a role in the prevention of the recurrence of cancerous lesions in the mouth, and also metastatic spread. A clinical trial under the auspices of the European Organization for Research and Treatment of Cancer was initiated in the early 1990s to investigate the possible preventive effect of vitamin A and N-acetylcyst-

eine (De Vries *et al.*, 1992). Other studies in this subject area have also been initiated (Lippman *et al.*, 1990, 1993; Toth *et al.*, 1993).

10.8 DATA FROM META-ANALYSIS

A major obstacle to be overcome in analytical studies of the aetiology of oral cancer is that of obtaining samples of sufficient size to enable the independent effects of several different variables to be adequately explained. One technique for overcoming the problem is meta-analysis, whereby, the data from a number of suitable studies are statistically combined in order to provide an investigation with much greater power than could be afforded by individual studies. A meta-analysis of oral cancer and associated factors, using data from three separate investigations, was conducted by Macfarlane (1993). The data were taken from studies conducted in New York State, Turin and Beijing (Marshall *et al.*, 1992; Merletti *et al.*, 1989, 1991; Zheng *et al.*, 1990a, b, 1993). The effects of alcohol, tobacco, daily intake of macronutrients (estimates of fat, protein and carbohydrate), and markers of fruit and vegetable consumption, indicating vitamin C and fibre intake, on the risk of oral cancer were analysed.

The results confirmed the independent effects of alcohol, tobacco and dietary factors in oral cancer aetiology. Also, the findings were generally consistent across the three centres and between genders. The investigation contained large enough numbers to analyse the risk in those who consumed only one of the two factors, alcohol or tobacco. In females there was an increased risk associated with both, although an effect from alcohol on its own could not be demonstrated in males. Dietary fibre and vitamin C intake were shown to be inversely associated with disease risk across the study populations after controlling for total energy (calorie) intake. The finding that the greatest reduction in risk in relation to high vitamin C intake occurred among heavy smokers, was considered to be of particular interest in the context of public health.

10.9 SUMMARY AND CONCLUSIONS

Variations in oral cancer incidence in different parts of the world suggest differential population exposures to specific risk factors. For example, high incidence rates in the Indian subcontinent are associated with the habit of chewing betel-quid and tobacco. There is strong evidence that tobacco smoking and high alcohol consumption are important independent risk factors for oral cancer. Moreover, their combined occurrence substantially increases the risk. The observed increases in intra-oral cancer in several Western countries, notably in adults under 60 years of age, may be related to raised alcohol consumption during the last 40 years since cigarette smoking has decreased.

A relationship suggesting a protective effect against oral cancer has been demonstrated from fruit and vegetable consumption. However, the problems of evaluating past dietary patterns and assessing the intake of individuals, and controlling for the confounding effects of alcohol intake and tobacco use, make valid studies in this area difficult to undertake.

11

ORAL SOFT TISSUE AND SALIVARY GLAND DISEASE

11.1 INTRODUCTION

The oral mucosa is the target organ for a number of disease processes. Atrophy of the buccal mucosa, as seen in response to nutritional deficiency or to ageing, can lead to thinning, loss of filiform papillae on the lingual mucosa with subsequent glossitis and sensitivity, and pain of the oral mucosa. Further thinning of the oral mucosa can lead to erosion or frank ulceration.

Separation of individual epithelial cells from one another, or from the underlying lamina propria, may lead to bulla formation, as is seen in vesiculo-bullous disorders. Thickening and hyperkeratosis of the oral mucosa can lead to whitening, resulting clinically in a white patch or leukoplakia. Finally, neoplastic change of the oral mucosa leads to the development of oral squamous cell carcinoma when dysplastic epithelium breaches the integrity of the basement membrane.

11.2 DISEASES OF THE SALIVARY GLAND

The salivary glands may enlarge as in sialosis, which may be due to protein malnutrition, diabetes mellitus, alcoholism, drugs, bulimia, or may be idiopathic. The salivary glands may also enlarge in autoimmune disease as seen in Sjögren's syndrome. The major salivary glands may also become virally infected as in mumps, or they may develop bacterial sialadenitis due to ascending infection from the mouth, particularly in patients with reduced salivary flow rate or mechanical blockage of the glands.

The glands may atrophy, either as a result of autoimmune disease, as in Sjögren's syndrome, due to an age-related change, or they may become atrophic as a result of radiotherapy or chemotherapy. In such cases xerostomia will result, leading to an increased risk of mucosal infection, particularly candidal infections, periodontal diseases and increased caries incidence. The use of certain drugs may also have a tem-porary effect on the production and flow rate of saliva. (Sneetny and Schwartg, 1986). The salivary glands are susceptible to a number of neoplastic processes which may be benign or malignant. The most common salivary gland tumour is the pleomorphic salivary adenoma.

11.3 INFLUENCE OF DIET AND NUTRITION

Disease results from the interaction of environmental and lifestyle factors against a genetic background. Increasingly, the importance of diet is being recognised. This is as true for oral mucosal disease as it is for systemic disease, although dietary changes and habits can influence both oral and systemic health. It is also increasingly evident that apart from the malnutrition still evident in parts of the developing world, suboptimal diets are widespread globally. This is a particular problem in elderly people because, although their energy needs fall with age, their nutrient needs are maintained or may even increase.

The importance of diet in relation to dental caries is well established, and widely appreciated. Nutrition can, however, also be important in relation to other oral diseases (Midda and Konig, 1994). Central to mucosal and periodontal integrity are adequate nutrition, and intact immune and other defences (such as saliva). Nutrient status is a major factor in the maintenance of normal immune responses.

Much disease, both systemic and oral, is more common in those of lower socioeconomic status (see Chapter 15). Malnutrition can impair oral mucosal health and immune defences: conversely oral mucosal disease can interfere with feeding and adequate nutrition status. Undernutrition is not the only problem; components of some diets may be harmful or indeed carcinogenic.

11.3.1 Fat, carbohydrate and protein intakes

There is no evidence that the amounts or types of fat intake has any beneficial or detrimental effects on the oral soft tissues or salivary glands. The level of carbohydrate intake also appears to have no direct impact on the oral soft tissues or salivary glands. However, diabetes mellitus, which may result in greater variation in blood glucose levels, is a risk factor for sialosis (Scully and Cawson, 1993).

Protein intake is more than adequate in the diets of most persons in the developed world. Severe protein energy malnutrition in the form of kwashiorkor, however, is associated with sialosis (Rauch and Gorlin, 1970). Also, protein deficiency can cause decreases in the immune response (Rosen and Geefhuysin, 1971; Mathur et al., 1972). In protein deficiency, smooth red glossitis, affecting particularly the anterior margins appears, and the tongue becomes scarlet. Angular cheilitis also may occur and may be associated with fissuring of the lower lip. In dark skinned races there may be loss of pigment along the vermilion border. These changes are probably due to tyrosine deficiency (Trowell et al., 1952; Van Wyck, 1965; Gillman, 1970).

11.3.2 Vitamins

Vitamins are required in only small amounts but inadequate intakes result in disease. Sometimes vitamin excess can also cause disease (Sauberlich and Machlin, 1992). Single vitamin deficiencies are very uncommon in industrialised countries, and indeed deficiency states occur rarely except through self neglect in special groups such as alcoholics and elderly people. The main food sources of the vitamins, along with the systemic and oral effects of deficiency, are shown in Table 11.1.

Precursors of vitamin A, and synthetic analogues such as the retinoic acids, can modulate epithelial cell differentiation of the oral mucosa. These were used in early studies to treat hyperkeratotic lesions of the oral mucosa (Smith, 1962; Silverman et al., 1963a, b; Ryssel et al., 1971; Günther, 1972a, b), and more recent studies have shown that retinoids such as 13-cis-retinoic acid (isotretinoin) and fenretinide, or carotenoids such as β-carotene, can suppress oral leukoplakias. Isotretinoin may also inhibit the development of carcinoma and can prevent second primary tumours in patients with oral squamous carcinomas (Scully and Boyle, 1992). There is evidence that 13-cis-retinoic acid (isotretinoin) and β-carotene enhance cell mediated immunity suggesting that immunomodulation, along with regulation of gene expression and antioxidant activity, can be protective mechanisms against tumour formation (Shklar and Schwartz, 1993).

A role for vitamin B_1 in burning mouth syndrome has been proposed (Foy et al., 1966), although others have not confirmed these findings (Bovina et al., 1969). Vitamins B_2 and B_6 have also been implicated in burning mouth syndrome (Lamey et al., 1986).

Glossitis and stomatitis have long been recognised in all forms of vitamin B_{12} deficiency (Barclay, 1851; Moller, 1851) which occurs clinically in 50–60% of patients with pernicious anaemia. The characteristic glossitis fluctuates in severity. Angular cheilitis has not been a regular feature of vitamin B_{12} deficiency (Ferguson, 1975) although recurrent oral ulceration is a feature (Wray et al., 1975). Oral changes in vitamin B_{12} deficiency occur rapidly and may be the only clinical evidence of disease. Following replacement therapy, symptoms are often relieved within 48 hours, and regeneration of lingual papillae occurs within four to seven days and may be normal within three weeks (Schieve and Rundles, 1949). Some patients may have a burning mouth even in the absence of recognisable mucosal disease (Wray et al., 1978). Vitamin B_{12} deficiency may also cause reversible dysplastic changes in the oral epithelium (Mitchell et al., 1986; Theaker and Porter, 1989).

The clinical and haematological effects of folate deficiency are virtually indistinguishable from B_{12} deficiency (Dreizen and Levy, 1969; Rose, 1971). Glossitis follows the same clinical and pathological patterns and recurrent aphthae are also frequent (Wray et al., 1975). Angular cheilitis is probably more common in folate deficiency, and is often exacerbated by secondary infection. Candidal infections are also more common in patients with folate deficiency, as is the case with vitamin B_{12} and iron deficiency (Jenkins et al., 1977). In common with vitamin B_{12} deficiency, replacement therapy using folic acid is usually attended by a prompt resolution of the oral signs (Wray et al., 1975). Recurrent aphthae have also been reported to respond to vitamin C replacement (Ferguson and Dagg, 1974). The salivary glands are also affected by vitamin C deficiency, and primary Sjögren's syndrome may develop (Hodges et al., 1970; Hood et al., 1970).

11.3.3 Trace elements

Trace elements are important to oral health, especially iron and zinc. The sources and effects of deficiency are shown in Table 11.2.

Table 11. 1 Vitamins: sources and effects of deficiency

Vitamin	Solubility	Food source	Deficiency syndrome	Oral signs of deficiency
A	Fat	Carotenoids (esp. β carotene): in carrots, dark green leafy vegetables, pumpkin, mango. Preformed vitamin A: in fish oils, liver, eggs, fortified margarine	Night blindness, xerophthalmia	Mucosal keratinisation, xerostomia, cheilitis, gingivitis
B_1	Water	Fortified wheat flour, fortified breakfast cereals, milk, eggs, yeast extract	Wernicke's encephalopathy	Oral sensitivity, mucosal vesicles, burning mouth syndrome
B_2	Water	Milk, cheese, eggs, fortified breakfast cereals, liver, kidney, whole grain cereals	Mucosal lesions	Angular cheilitis, glossitis, recurrent aphthae, bluish discolouration, sialorrhoea
Niacin	Water	Liver, kidney, milk, cheese, eggs, beef, chicken, pork, yeast extract, instant coffee, peas, beans	Pellagra	Mucosal atrophy, angular cheilitis
B_6	Water	Liver, meat, fish, whole grain cereals, milk, peanuts	Glossitis; neuropathy	Glossitis, cheilitis, burning mouth syndrome, ulceration, lip fissures
B_{12}	Water	Meat, fish, eggs, milk, cheese, fortified breakfast cereal	Megaloblastosis; neuropathies; mucosal lesions	Glossitis, stomatitis, recurrent aphthae, dysplasia, angular cheilitis
Folate	Water	Liver, kidney, green leafy vegetables, peas, beans, oranges, fortified breads and breakfast cereals	Megaloblastosis; mucosal lesions	Glossitis, stomatitis, recurrent aphthae, angular cheilitis
C	Water	Citrus fruits, potatoes, green vegetables, fortified fruit drinks	Scurvy	Recurrent aphthae, angular cheilitis, periodontitis
D	Fat	Fortified milk, fatty fish, fortified margarine, eggs, fatty meat	Rickets; osteomalacia	None
E	Fat	Vegetable oils, wholegrain cereals, nuts, eggs, fortified margarine	None	None
K	Fat	Vegetables, peas, beans, liver	Hypo-prothrombinaemia and bleeding tendency.	Gingival bleeding, post-extraction haemorrhage

Oral manifestations of iron deficiency are particularly prominent (Waldenström, 1938; Beveridge et al., 1965; Rose, 1968; Rennie et al., 1984). In a large series of iron deficient patients, atrophic glossitis was found in 39% of patients and angular cheilitis in 14%, and these changes may occur before the development of anaemia (Waldenström, 1938; Rustung, 1949). The severity of the glossitis does not approach that seen in vitamin B_{12} deficiency or folate deficiency, although in severe cases there is redness and atrophy of the filiform and fungiform papillae with marked thinning of the epithelium (Taft et al., 1958; Baird et al., 1961). There are similar changes in the buccal mucosa but these occur less frequently (Jacobs, 1960). Recurrent aphthae may also be associated with an iron deficient state which responds to replacement therapy (Wray et al., 1975).

In the classic description of iron deficiency,

Table 11. 2 Trace elements: sources and effects of deficiency

Nutrient	Food source	Deficiency syndrome	Oral signs of deficiency
Iron	Meat, fish, vegetables, fortified bread and breakfast cereals	Anaemia Koilonychia Kelly-Paterson syndrome	Glossitis, angular cheilitis, mucosal atrophy, candidosis
Zinc	Shellfish, fish, meat, poultry, dairy foods, pulses	Developmental retardation Acrodermatitis enteropathica	Geographic tongue Taste disturbance

dysphagia and post-cricoid oesophageal stricture was made by Kelly and by Paterson in 1919, and subsequently by Vincent in 1922. Post-cricoid dysphagia has been found in about 7% of iron deficient subjects (Beveridge *et al.*, 1965). The neoplastic potential of the Kelly-Paterson syndrome may have been overestimated in the past and subsequent prospective studies show a lower incidence (Owen, 1950; Shammas and Benedict, 1958; Jones, 1961; Chisholm *et al.*, 1971).

Zinc deficiency may lead to defective collagen synthesis and is also involved in taste. Taste disturbance is associated with zinc deficiency, and geographic tongue has also been reported to respond to zinc replacement therapy (Gibson *et al.*, 1990). Zinc therapy has been shown to be ineffective in the management of recurrent aphthous stomatitis (Wray, 1982).

12

THE FETUS

12.1 FIRST TRIMESTER OF PREGNANCY

12.1.1 Embryogenesis and organogenesis

In the first few weeks of pregnancy, during the stage of embryogenesis, the primitive oral epithelium bulges into the underlying mesenchyme at various places to form knob-like swellings surrounded by vascular tissue. These are the tooth buds, and the buds of the front teeth including the incisors, canines and first molars are formed first. The epithelial tissue becomes the enamel organ and the mesenchyme tissue goes on to form the papilla. Dentine comes from the dental papilla; cells from the dental papilla differentiate to form cells called odontoblasts. Enamel formation begins at about 14 weeks post conception in the primary incisors and is completed about 14 weeks after birth (Lunt and Law, 1974). By the fourteenth week of pregnancy, most other organs in the fetus have formed and are recognisable as heart, kidneys, limbs etc, but their microscopic structure is still quite different from that seen in later life. A chronology of tooth development in the fetus is shown in Table 12.1.

The well-known nutritional insults at this stage of pregnancy, which can interfere with 'organogenesis' in humans, are folate deficiency or vitamin A excess. Both nutrient insults can adversely affect the development of the central nervous system, causing neural tube defects involving abnormalities of the brain, spinal cord and surrounding bone. The children thus affected are not described as having any dental or oral abnormalities.

12.2 SECOND AND THIRD TRIMESTER OF PREGNANCY

12.2.1 Histiogenesis

This stage of development, i.e. the formation of individual tissues in an organ and a maturation of the microscopic appearances, continues throughout pregnancy and for some organs into postnatal life.

The development of the enamel may be regarded as a form of histiogenesis. The enamel initially forms a 'cap' on the tooth bud and then spreads down in a 'bell' around the developing tooth. The process of enamel development consists of the formation of an organic matrix and then a process of mineralisation with crystals of apatite (Nylen, 1964).

Nutritional and other insults during either organic matrix formation or mineralisation will lead to hypoplasia of the enamel with pitting, furrowing, or an abnormal appearance. Matrix formation could in theory be affected by a whole variety of nutritional deficiencies or excesses affecting connective tissue such as vitamins C, A and many trace elements. There is little evidence of the effects of these micronutrient deficiencies *in utero* on tooth development in humans. In rats, vitamin A deficiency induced in the dams led to deficiency in the pups, with dentine and enamel abnormalities and higher caries scores when the teeth erupted (Harris and Navia, 1980). There is, however, some circumstantial evidence in humans implicating vitamin D deficiency during pregnancy, in the aetiology of hypomineralisation and hypoplasia of the developing enamel.

12.2.2 Hypocalcaemia and vitamin D deficiency

Three studies in Britain have shown enamel hypoplasia in the primary dentition to be common in children who, around the age of 7–14 days of postnatal life, experienced an abnormally low plasma calcium, i.e. those who had late neonatal hypocalcaemia (defined as levels below 1.8 mmol/l) (Stimmler *et al.*, 1973: 12 children; Purvis *et al.*, 1973: 63 children; Levine and Keen, 1974: 15 children). The two latter papers included histology of the shed teeth.

At the time of these studies, late neonatal hypocalcaemia was partly a reflection of the very high phosphate intake of bottle-fed babies, who received cows' milk rather than modified infant formulas which were not widely used in Britain until 1975, but some relationship to the vitamin

Table 12.1   Intrauterine chronology of tooth development

Tooth		Tooth germ fully formed	Dentine formation begins
Deciduous	Incisors Canines 1st molars 2nd molars	3–4 months fetal life	4–6 month fetal life
Permanent	Incisors	30th week fetal life	3–4 months (upper lateral incisors 10–12 months)
	Canines	30th week fetal life	4–5 months
	Premolars	30th week fetal life	$1\frac{1}{2}$–$2\frac{1}{2}$ years
	1st molars	24th week fetal life	Birth

Source: from Hogan (1995).

D status of mothers was also apparent (Dent and Gupta, 1975). The enamel hypoplasia described was unlikely to have been caused by such a short period of hypocalcaemia which was quickly reversed by treatment. Attention turned, therefore, to the possible influences of the intrauterine environment.

Purvis et al., (1973) showed that the incidence of neonatal hypocalcaemia in Edinburgh was seasonal, and related to fewer hours of sunshine during the third trimester of the pregnancy. They presumed it to be an effect of lack of maternal vitamin D. Histology of shed incisors from five children also suggested the enamel hypoplasia dated from the third trimester, although Levine and Keen (1974) disputed this conclusion. Mellander et al. (1982) have also shown a higher prevalence of enamel hypoplasia in infants born in the winter months in Goteborg; 20 out of 27 cases were born between October and March. This association was not found in the more recent Boston study of Needleman et al. (1992). Interestingly, Boston is many miles further south than Sweden or Scotland, so there was probably less seasonal variation in solar irradiation.

In a later intervention study in Edinburgh, Cockburn et al., (1980) showed that vitamin D supplements in pregnancy led to a fall in the incidence of neonatal hypocalcaemia (6% compared with 13% in controls) and in enamel hypoplasia (7% in the supplement group of 30 compared with 48% in the unsupplemented group of 31 who had experienced hypocalcaemia). Other studies have shown the effect of vitamin D supplements in pregnancy in the prevention of neonatal hypocalcaemia, but have not reported on the children's teeth.

The exact mechanism by which maternal vitamin D deficiency results in enamel hypoplasia is unclear. Cockburn et al. (1980) speculated that a compensatory maternal hyperparathyroidism during pregnancy played a role.

12.2.3 Intrauterine growth

During the second and third trimesters of pregnancy the fetus grows rapidly in size and the processes of histiogenesis continue.

A baby is described as 'preterm' if born before 37 weeks gestation (normal gestation is about 40 weeks). A preterm baby who has grown satisfactorily will have a weight 'appropriate for gestational age'. A simplified interpretation is that growth was progressing satisfactorily until some acute process led to early labour. Preterm babies will usually have a low birthweight because they have been born early. Low birthweight is classified as less than 2500 g. Babies who have not grown well in utero will have a weight below that expected for the gestational age, i.e. they are light or small for gestational age. They also have a low birthweight, but because they have not grown satisfactorily in utero. Light-for-gestational-age babies are sometimes described as having had 'intrauterine malnutrition', but growth restricted may be a better description, since being light for gestational age has many causes, e.g. maternal smoking, hypertension and under-nutrition.

What happens to tooth development with these different patterns of intrauterine growth? Needleman et al., (1992) summarised a number of previous studies in relation to enamel defects (Table 12.2). In some of the studies it is not possible to define the intrauterine growth patterns in the way described above but some general conclusions can be drawn.

● Preterm delivery is associated with a higher prevalence of enamel defects—about 45% affected—compared to less than 15% in those born at term (comparison of lines 1, 2; 13, 14; 18, 19; 37, 38). It is unclear whether, or not, very preterm babies have more enamel defects than moderately preterm ones.

Table 12.2 Prevalences of enamel defects of primary teeth in preterm and/or low birthweight infants

	Sample		Children affected (%)			References
	N	Criteria	Hypoplasia	Opacity	Total	
1	16	<7th month GA			50.0	Stein (1947)
2	>200	AGA			<1.0	
3	99	P			56.6	Forrester and Miller (1955)
4	109	AGA			3.7	Miller and Forrester (1959)
5	68	<3000 g			32.4	Grahnen & Larson (1958)
6	61	>3000 g			13.1	
7	21	<2300 g	23.8			Rosenwieg & Sahar (1962)
8	80	>2300 g	1.2			
9	26	SGA, normal length			0.0	Grahnen et al (1972)
10	26	SGA, short			19.2	
11	26	Dysmature			11.5	
12	56	AGA, normal weight			12.5	
13	82	<38 wks	21.9	20.7	42.6	* Grahnen et al. (1974)
14	39	AGA	5.1	10.3	15.4	
15	64	P & <200 g	26.6	18.7	45.3	Rosentein (1974)
16	20	SGA	20.0			Funakoshi et al. (1981)
17	32	AGA	34.4			
18	29	<34 wks	41.4	*		
19	23	>34 wks	13.0			
20	91	>2000 g	20.9	12.1	33.0	Mellander et al. (1982)
21	48	AGA	16.7	22.9	39.6	
22	53	PAGA			37.7	
23	25	PSGA			16.0	*
24	13	AGA & SGA			23.1	
25	67	<1500 g	20.8	31.4	52.2	* Johson et al. (1984)
26	46	AGA	4.3	21.7	26.0	
27	91	<2000 g	17.6	12.1	29.7	Noren et al. (1984)
28	48	FAGA	16.7	22.9	39.6	
29	63	<1500 g			60.3	Seow et al. (1984)
30	106	<37 wks & <1500 g	37.0			Pimlott et al. (1985)
31	77	<1500 g	51.9	10.4	62.3	* Seow et al. (1987)
32	33	1500–2500 g	21.2	6.1	27.3	*
33	47	>2500 g	6.4	6.4	12.7	
34	45	1149 + 191 g, 29.4 + 2.3 wks			68.9	Seow et al. (1989)
35	110	<2000 g	71.0	22.0	77.0	* Fearne et al. (1990)
36	93	>2000 g	15.0	27.0	37.0	
37	19	<37 wks	42.1	*		Needleman et al. (1991)
38	433	>37 wks	17.6			
39	22	<2500 g	40.9	*		
40	430	>2500 g	17.4			

Key:
A: appropriate; GA: gestational age; H: hypoplasia; S: small; F: full term; P: preterm; AGA: appropriate weight for gestational age; SGA: small or light for gestational age.
$*p < 0.05$.
Source: Needleman (1992).

- Retarded intrauterine growth may be associated with a higher prevalence of enamel defects, but if there is an effect, it is less than the effect of preterm delivery, and in only one study was the observed differences statistically significant—20–37% affected compared to 13–20% in those who were an appropriate weight for gestational age (comparison of lines 10, 12; 16, 17; 22, 23).
- Low birthweight babies, who may be preterm or light-for-gestational age, have a higher prevalence of enamel defects. Figures are very variable: 23–77% affected compared to 1–37% in babies of normal weight (comparison of lines 5, 6; 7, 8; 35, 36; 39, 40).

The evidence concerning low birthweight babies, where gestational age is not specified, does not help to differentiate the effect of being born early as opposed to poor intrauterine growth, and for the purposes of trying to detect intrauterine influences on dental development, should probably be ignored. Pragmatically, however, it does indicate that all low birthweight babies require extra dental supervision in the early years of life.

The higher prevalence of enamel defects in preterm babies of appropriate weight for gestation may have been due to intrauterine factors, but it seems these possible factors were insufficient to retard growth. It seems as likely, therefore, that the effect on teeth was postnatal and related to the various problems which preterm babies are more prone to in early life, e.g. hypoxia, infection and some nutritional problems.

The association of dental defects with intrauterine growth retardation is weak. In the study of Needleman et al. (1992), the increased prevalence of enamel hypoplasia in small-for-gestational-age babies did not reach statistical significance ($p = 0.09$). A recent London study showed no higher prevalence of enamel defects in children who had been born light-for-gestational age (Brook et al., 1997). Grahnen et al. (1972) concluded intrauterine under-nutrition does not seem to be an important factor in the aetiology of clinically demonstrable enamel mineralisation defects of primary teeth. Perhaps this conclusion should be modified to indicate that intrauterine malnutrition causing growth retardation is not closely related to enamel defects.

12.3 INTRAUTERINE DEFICIENCIES AND DENTAL CARIES

It is unclear whether dental caries is more likely to develop, or become serious, in teeth with en-

amel hypoplasia. Stimmler et al., (1973), in their study of 12 children with hypoplasia following neonatal hypocalcaemia, also commented on the advanced caries many of them had. On the other hand, Bramstedt (1975) reviewing the results of various studies in humans and rats, concluded that changes in the mineral composition of teeth had no relation to the development of caries.

There is some evidence of a greater susceptibility to caries in rats born to dams that had been experimentally undernourished during pregnancy and early lactation. Alvarez and Navia (1989) reviewing this evidence, based mainly on work in Birmingham USA, made the following points:

The offspring of rats that were fed a low-protein, high-sucrose diet grew more slowly and their molars erupted later and were significantly smaller than those of the control animals (Holloway et al., 1961). If rats are undernourished during the time that molars are being formed, and they are fed a moderate caries-promoting diet, they will develop 50% higher caries scores than adequately fed control offspring fed the same caries-promoting diet (Shaw et al., 1963). A moderate protein deficiency imposed during the period of tooth development in rats was accompanied by diminished growth of incisors and molars and by delayed eruption of their teeth. Protein-energy malnutrition affected salivary flow and composition (Diorio et al., 1973; Meneker and Navia, 1973). Protein-energy malnutrition imposed on rat dams during lactation increased acid solubility of the enamel of molars from rat pups suckling from these dams (Aponte-Merced and Navia, 1980). Vitamin A deficiency during tooth development was also associated with changes in dentine formation and increased susceptibility to caries (Harris and Navia, 1980).

It is difficult to know, however, to what extent these observations are relevant to the human. Also the period of dietary restriction in some of the experiments was postnatal as well as in utero. Similar comments may be made concerning the greater susceptibility to caries found in the offspring of rats with suboptimal zinc nutrition during pregnancy and lactation (Cerklewski, 1981).

12.4 SUMMARY AND CONCLUSIONS

Despite suggestive work in rats linking fetal nutrition to dental development and susceptibility to caries, evidence in humans is less convincing. The known nutritional teratogenic influences in early human pregnancy do not appear to interfere with the development of the tooth bud. Fetal growth restriction in later pregnancy, may be associated with a modest increase in the prevalence of enamel hypoplasia. Low birthweight babies, whether preterm or light, for, gestational age, require extra dental surveillance. Both association and intervention studies suggest that maternal vitamin D deficiency leads to enamel hypoplasia in the primary dentition. It is unclear whether, or not, enamel hypoplasia increases the susceptibility to caries. Vitamin D deficiency is more common in the northern parts of the country, in Asian people living in Britain, and in those living in innercity areas. These groups all have a higher prevalence of caries. In recent years the prevalence of overt vitamin D deficiency has declined, and the prevalence of caries has also fallen. This secular change is considered to be mainly due to fluoride in water and/or toothpaste. A speculation is that improved vitamin D nutrition *in utero* could also have played a role in the reduction in caries of the primary dentition. Current policy is that a pregnant woman should receive a vitamin D supplement (approximately 10 ug daily), unless her professional adviser is confident that alternative sources from sun and diet are reasonable. This recommendation is particularly important for women living in the northern parts of the country, and women from the Indian subcontinent.

13

INFANTS AND CHILDREN

13.1 INTRODUCTION

The oral disease that has the greatest influence on the quality of life for children living in the UK is dental caries. Despite the remarkable reduction in the prevalence of caries in children over the last quarter of a century (see Chapter 5), in 1993 there were still 45% of 5-year-old children affected by the disease with a mean number of 1.7 diseased teeth, and 40% still had some untreated decay (O'Brien, 1994). Among these young children, 12% had already experienced tooth extraction, mostly under general anaesthesia. By the age of 16 years, about two-thirds (68%) of the UK population had experience of the disease and over half (56%) had to have teeth extracted (O'Brien, 1994). By the age of 5 years, tooth extraction under general anaesthesia is the first experience of surgery for many children and this is carried out, for the most part, away from the protective environment of a paediatric hospital. In England in 1992/93, over 260,000 general anaesthetics were given to patients under the age of 18 years for tooth extraction (NWRHA, 1994). The effects of tooth extraction on both the young children and their families have been clearly documented in a survey conducted by Bridgman (1993). For many adults, the fear of dental treatment still lies in unpleasant memories of treatment received when they were very young.

The incidence of disease remaining precludes the ability of traditional treatment services to answer the problem (Downer, 1994). Curzon and Pollard (1997) have suggested that £66 would be an appropriate annual capitation fee for the treatment of children, making a total of some £800 million for the whole UK child population, or approximately the entire tax payers' contribution to the general dental services. Added to financial aspects, the social cost of children missing school and parents' time in gaining treatment for their children, and the emotional cost to both, must be considered.

It is clear that dental caries is an important health problem in the UK, affecting some groups of children more seriously than others, and that its solution cannot be left entirely in the hands of dentists to provide treatment for the disease that occurs.

13.2 INFANTS AND PRE-SCHOOL CHILDREN

13.2.1 Dental caries

Few comprehensive studies had been made of the levels of caries among pre-school children until the National Diet and Nutrition Survey of children from 1.5–4.5 years of age was carried out (Hinds and Gregory, 1995). This showed that dental decay was a considerable problem even before school age, with 17% of these children already suffering the disease, rising from 4% at 1.5–2.5 years to 30% at 3.5–4.5 years. Overall, 2% of these children had teeth extracted because of decay and only 2% of the remaining decay was treated.

A north–south gradient in experience of the disease existed in all age groups, with infants in Scotland having higher levels than those in the south of England (Figure 13.1). More of the disease was also discovered in children of poorer families and those whose mothers were less well educated.

In this study, 95% of the parents completed a record of the weighed dietary intake of their children over a four-day period; they also completed a food frequency questionnaire. Particular interest was shown in the relationship between dental health and feeding patterns.

Most children (87%) were reported to have used a feeding bottle at some time from birth; even at the age of 1.5–2.5 years, half (49%) were using a bottle and 8% of the 3.5–4.5 year age group were still using bottles. Within the bottle, more than half had milk and one-quarter had drinks containing sugars, such as squashes, carbonated drinks and flavoured milk drinks.

A higher proportion of those below the age of

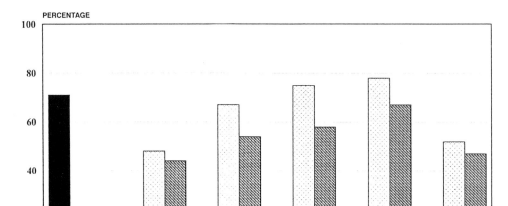

Figure 13.1 Children's dental health surveys. Prevalence of 5-years-olds with decay, by region of the UK.
Source: O'Brien (1994). © Crown Copyright. Reproduced with permission: Office for National Statistics.

3.5 years who were reported to have a drink in bed at night had decay, compared to those who did not; 21% compared with 12% who never had a drink in bed (Figure 13.2). In 3.5–4.5-year-olds, differences were not statistically significant.

Among all children who were reported to consume drinks in bed every night, 29% who had a sugary drink had experienced decay compared with 11% who only had milk.

There was a strong relationship between the reported average weekly household expenditure on confectionery and dental decay. In the oldest age band, 20% of those where less than £2 per week was spent on sweets and confectionery had decay, but this rose to 60% where weekly expenditure was in excess of £5. Fewer non-manual households reported spending more than £5 per week on chocolates and sweets on average, than manual households. For all ages, 43% of children had confectionery and 24% had carbonated drinks most days. The proportions rose with increasing age.

Half the children (49%) were reported to have started toothbrushing before the age of one year and, of these, less than 1% used a non-fluoride toothpaste. The younger the age at which brushing was claimed to begin, and the more fre-

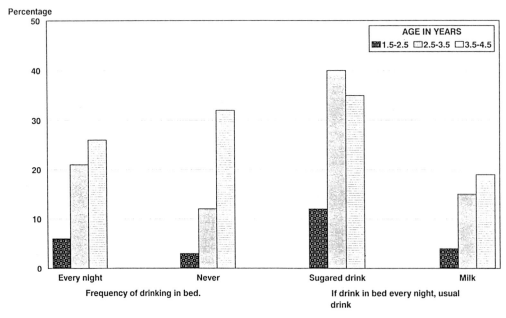

Figure 13.2 Proportion of children with any decay experience by age and night-time drinking practices.
Source: Hinds and Gregory (1995). © Crown Copyright. Reproduced with permission: Office for National Statistics.

quently it was said to be performed, the lower the proportion having tooth decay. Those children where an adult was said to assist with brushing also had less decay.

Dental decay was lowest among infrequent consumers of sugar confectionery and carbonated drinks who had their teeth brushed most often, and highest among children who were frequent consumers of such food and drink and who brushed their teeth least frequently. Frequent toothbrushing did not seem to completely outweigh the damaging effects of the frequent consumption of sugars.

After controlling for the effects of the main discriminators between decay experience for the different age groups, further independent relationships with caries levels included, for 2.5–3.5-year-olds, usually having a drink containing sugar at bedtime. For 3.5–4.5-year-olds, in descending order of importance were, the region in which they lived, household expenditure on confectionery and whether their parents were in receipt of Income Support or Family Credit.

In infancy, breast milk, infant formula and the follow-on milks are the major sources of nutrition. Babies should ideally be breast-fed for the first few months of life, but eventually many infants will be offered feeds from a baby bottle. Breast milk contains 'milk sugar' or lactose, the least cariogenic of the sugars, at approximately 7 g/100 ml. Milk, either from the breast or an infant formula in a bottle, is a baby's staple diet in the early months. Casein-dominant infant formulas and follow-on milks contain calcium and phosphorus which may help to reduce enamel dissolution as does the protein casein. This has the ability to buffer or neutralise the acid produced in plaque (Moynihan, 1995). It has also been suggested that components of milk fat help to lower its cariogenicity. Thus, although milk and milk products contain lactose, the other properties of milk seem more than adequate to protect the teeth from decay. Studies have shown that cow's milk does not reduce the pH of dental plaque below a level necessary to produce enamel dissolution (Rugg-Gunn et al., 1985).

'Nursing-bottle caries' is a condition in which the upper anterior deciduous teeth and, in more severe cases, the deciduous molars become carious. This type of caries is normally associated with ad libitum bottle-feeding, particularly at night. In developed countries, the prevalence is reported to be between 1–12% (Milnes, 1996). This may be higher in non-industrialised countries and among the disadvantaged in industrialised countries. It causes pain and infection and leads to the early extraction of these teeth with

the possible *sequelae* of inadequate function, loss of space for the permanent teeth and speech and psychosocial problems (Brice et al., 1996). Nursing-bottle caries most frequently arises because the infant is allowed to suck liquids containing sugars from the bottle for prolonged periods, particularly while asleep, when the rate of flow of saliva is considerably reduced. The same may result from including sugar containing liquids in a reservoir feeder or dipping a dummy into a sugary syrup (Winter, 1980). In order to minimise the risk of this scenario, it is recommended that babies begin to drink from a cup from the age of six months, and that from the age of one year they should be discouraged from using a bottle altogether (DH, 1994). When babies are bottle-feeding, the bottle should be held by an adult. The practice of allowing a child to hold a bottle, or of propping the bottle on the baby's pillow, should be avoided.

In rare cases, a pattern of caries similar to nursing-bottle caries has been seen with prolonged breast-feeding (Roberts, 1982). Once again, it arises when the baby is allowed to sleep with the nipple still in its mouth.

Some mothers are advised to feed their babies soya infant formulae for medical reasons, e.g. an allergy to cow's milk protein or because of a metabolic disorder. Soya infant formulae contain glucose syrups derived from hydrolysed starch, instead of lactose, which has led to concerns that they may be more cariogenic. Although Moynihan et al. (1996) could find no difference in acidogenicity between a soya and a milk formula, good feeding and weaning practices are still necessary in this group of infants. The cariogenicity of these formulae will vary according to their mode of consumption. Healthy children can drink cow's milk at one year, but those with an intolerance to cow's milk may not, thus remaining on soya formulae for a longer time. These formulae have more carbohydrate than cow's milk and contain lower concentrations of protective factors such as calcium and phosphorus.

13.2.2 Tooth-tissue loss

There is increasing concern among paediatric dentists and dental epidemiologists that the prevalence and severity of tooth-tissue loss is increasing in the young. Because of the lack of comparable longitudinal population studies, however, this hypothesis cannot yet be verified. The National Diet and Nutrition Survey of infants and pre-school children (Hinds and Gregory, 1995) showed the prevalence of this condition to be 13% in those aged 3.5–4.5 years of age.

Although tooth-tissue loss when confined only to enamel is sometimes difficult to diagnose, once dentine is involved, the condition becomes clinically more apparent. Thus, by 5–6 years of age, a quarter of the children examined showed tooth-tissue loss involving dentine or even the pulp (O'Brien, 1994). Loss of enamel or even some dentine seldom requires treatment in these young children, for the teeth are shed before any serious effects result. However, in the few that are so severely affected that the pulps of the anterior teeth are exposed leading to their infection and the need for extraction, the condition can cause much distress and disfigurement.

There are three specific types of tooth-tissue loss due to mechanisms other than dental caries (Imfeld, 1996) (see Chater 7). Erosion results from chemical attack of the enamel by acids other than those produced by plaque bacteria. Attrition is caused by mastication or contact between the occlusal or approximal surfaces of teeth. Abrasion, which is a more important factor in adults, results from mechanical factors other than those involved in attrition or erosion. Often two or more of these types of wear occur together and it may be difficult to differentiate between them (Nunn, 1996) but the site of the wear, its appearance and particularly a detailed history of associated factors, will help in determining the likely aetiology. Tooth wear is irreversible and, therefore, its severity increases with age.

The pH levels of some baby fruit juices and drinks intended to be drunk undiluted are approximately 3.5, and diluting them 10-fold only raised this to about pH4, still below the critical value for demineralising the tooth surface (Smith and Shaw, 1987). Many of these drinks have a high titratable acidity making it difficult for the saliva to rapidly neutralise them (Duggal and Curzon, 1989). It is possible that, if these juices are held in contact with the teeth for prolonged periods of time, for example, in feeding bottles or reservoir feeders, they will contribute materially to tooth-tissue loss in infants and toddlers. Vitamin C preparations and some iron tonics fed to young children also have low pH levels.

Persistent vomiting is another cause of tooth-tissue loss. In most young children symptoms of oesophageal reflux resolve by 18 months, although resolution may not be lifelong (Booth, 1992). Children with cerebral palsy may have persistent gastric reflux although vomiting may not be a feature. Little is known of the incidence or prevalence of gastro-oesophageal reflux in the young.

13.3 SCHOOL CHILDREN

13.3.1 Dental caries

In the UK, there have been three dental surveys of school children conducted by the Office of Population Censuses and Surveys (OPCS). The most recent (O'Brien, 1994), showed that the declining levels of dental caries recorded in the two earlier studies was continuing, if at a slower rate (Figure 13.3). However, there is concern that the levelling off in decay rates in 5-year-old children may conceal an increase among some groups of the population. In some parts of the country, caries experience at 5 years of age has shown a small increase (Downer, 1994).

Despite the general improvement in the dental health of children over the last quarter of a century, there is still a marked geographic gradient in its prevalence, with the lowest levels in the south and the highest in Scotland and Northern Ireland. Caries also seems to be polarising, largely among the less advantaged groups in society. For example, in Glasgow the mean caries experience at the age of 12 years was 2.7, while in the more affluent city of Edinburgh only 45 km away, it was only 1.4 (Downer et al., 1994). It has long been recognised that dental caries is related to social class and there is evidence to show that children from deprived backgrounds have the greatest need for dental care (Pitts, 1997).

13.3.2. Tooth-tissue loss

Tooth-tissue loss in the permanent dentition of young people is less common and less severe than in the deciduous teeth. At the age of 15 years, 27% of the population showed evidence of the condition, but only in 1% had this progressed to expose the dentine (O'Brien, 1994).

The frequent consumption of citrus fruits is a well documented cause of tooth-tissue loss, and other acidic foods such as yoghurts and foods pickled in vinegar may also be implicated. More recently, the excessive consumption of acid drinks has been suggested as a cause (Jarvinen et al., 1991; Figure 13.4).

Tooth-tissue loss is also associated with the eating disorder bulimia nervosa, and sometimes anorexia nervosa, as a result of vomiting (Robb et al., 1995). Both these conditions predominantly affect females in industrialised countries

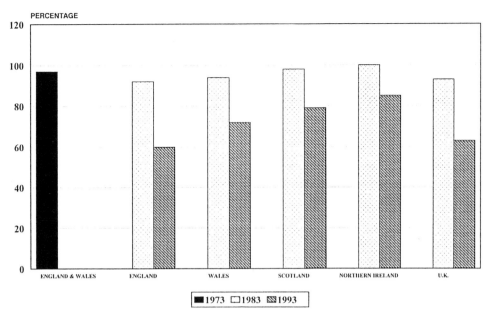

Figure 13.3 Children's dental health surveys. Proportions of 15-years-olds with decay, by region of the UK. Source: O'Brien (1994). © Crown Copyright. Reproduced with permission: Office for National Statistics.

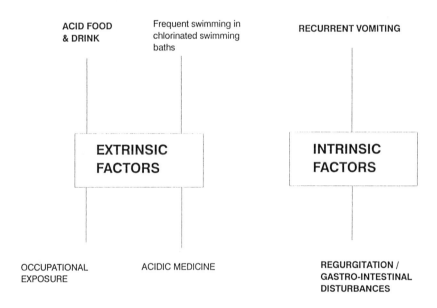

Figure 13.4 Aetiology of erosion.

and begin in adolescence. In a South Australian adolescent population, the prevalence of anorexia nervosa was measured as 0.1–0.2% (Bentovim and Morton, 1990), and it is almost certainly lower in younger children.

Tooth-tissue loss is potentially disfiguring. Teeth appear more yellow and anterior teeth can look fractured in the more advanced cases. Function is affected as the teeth may become sensitive to thermal stimuli. The costly treatment needed to repair the damage is contra-indicated until the causes have been found and corrected.

13.3.3 Chronically ill and disadvantaged children

Although dental caries causes much suffering among the many healthy children that it affects, its influence rarely causes serious morbidity. However, there are many disadvantaged children whose health, or even life, is put at risk by the sequelae of dental caries or its treatment. Chronically sick children, such as those with blood disorders, long-term chest complaints and renal disease, must avoid focal infection, the need for tooth extraction or the risks that go with general anaesthesia (Hobson, 1980). Intellectually or physically disadvantaged children may also be at risk from aspects of dental treatment (Shaw, 1997; Nunn, 1997). Although modern techniques by specialist dentists often help reduce these risks (Meechan and Welbury, 1996), the more obvious course is to avoid the disease altogether. It is important that their parents, carers and those health professionals who assist them, appreciate the need to exercise on their behalf the sensible use of sugar and the effective application of fluoride (Brown, 1980).

13.4 THE CONTROL OF DENTAL CARIES IN THE YOUNG

13.4.1 Sugar consumption in children

The most important dietary factor in the aetiology of dental caries is the consumption of sugars, with the frequency of consumption a particularly important influence. Since young people are eating more snacks, and mealtimes together are becoming less a feature of family life, it is important to provide snacks for children that are free from sugar. The eating patterns of young people have been characterised as a tendency to skip meals, especially breakfast, to consume large amounts of snack foods and drinks and to engage in frequent attempts at dieting. These practices pose a threat to both general and dental health.

In terms of the social influences on young people's patterns of food consumption, there are key factors at various stages of development. At the infant and toddler stage, the innate food preferences are strongly influenced by the social learning experiences of the child's mother. Once school starts, peer group pressure becomes an increasingly powerful influence and that of the family diminishes. This pattern becomes even stronger during adolescence. In a qualitative study of the meaning of foods among adolescent girls, Chapman and Maclean (1993) showed a conflict between adults and children regarding food; 'junk foods' were associated in their minds with pleasure, friends, weight gain and growing independence while 'healthy foods' were heavily associated with family values.

Holt (1991) found that nearly all 4-year-old children in her study had one or more sugar-containing snacks or drinks on most days. Mean caries scores were higher with increasing numbers of intakes. It was concluded that snacks are part of the eating pattern of young children and the most popular items contained added sugar.

If snacking must be accepted as part of the dietary culture of young people, then the consumption of snacks that are least harmful to the teeth should be emphasised. Thus, fresh fruit is to be recommended as relatively safe, and cheese may even have properties that protect the teeth (Rugg-Gunn et al., 1975). Grenby (1990) showed that peanuts and most crisps have little or no cariogenic potential, but some varieties of crisps, such as cheese and onion flavour and some with special shapes, were comparable to semi-sweet biscuits containing 22% total sugars. In offering advice on dentally acceptable snacks, he concluded that it is safer to recommend savoury rather than sweetened products and, of the former, the less processed varieties seem to offer less of a cariogenic challenge. Cooked staple foods such as potatoes and bread are of low cariogenicity.

Sugary foods and drinks are best confined to meal times, and milk and water are the most appropriate between meal drinks, as they do not contain dentally harmful sugars.

An interest has developed recently in confectionery that contain bulk sweeteners such as xylitol or isomaltitol in place of sugar. These 'tooth-friendly sweets' have a useful role, particularly where dietary advice to reduce sweet snacks is difficult to achieve (British Society of Paediatric Dentistry, 1995). However, in 1991 the sugar-free sector of the UK confectionery market was worth only £6 million (where total sales for confectionery exceeded £4 billion) (Pike, 1994).

Chewing gum, especially the sugar-free variety, can also be recommended as safe for teeth. Those containing xylitol may even partially protect the teeth from caries (Makinen et al., 1995).

The quantity and frequency of sugar consumption is related to the level of caries in a population. It has been recommended that the population average intake of non-milk extrinsic sugars should not exceed 10% of total energy intake (DH, 1991), but the average intake in children aged 1.5–2.5 years is 17% and at 3.5–4.5 years is 20% (Hinds and Gregory, 1995).

In the report 'Easy to Swallow, Hard to Stomach' (National Food Alliance, 1995) the nature and extent of food advertising on television aimed at children and adolescents was examined and compared with that aimed at adults. Monitoring was carried out over two separate weeks. Advertisements for food and soft drinks accounted for seven out of ten advertisements on children's weekday television programmes, with only two out of ten being targeted at adults after 9.30 pm. Foods high in fat, sugar and salt accounted for 80–100% of all food advertising on children's television (Nelson, 1993). Of the accounted for 80–100% of all food advertising on children's television (Nelson, 1993). Of the 549 adverts monitored, only two were for fruit and vegetables. It would seem more appropriate to direct such advertising towards adults rather than children.

13.4.2 The influence of fluoride

The appropriate use of fluoride is fundamental in the control of dental caries. In the UK, the two most important vehicles for bringing the benefits of fluoride to the child population are water and toothpaste. Unfortunately, only some 10% of the UK population currently receives water containing fluoride at the optimal level of 1 ppm. Studies have shown that this will reduce the level of caries in children by at least 50% (Murray et al., 1991; Jones et al., 1997). It also makes dramatic reductions in the proportion of children experiencing toothache, needing extractions under general anaesthesia, and those with the highly destructive form of the disease where the whole dentition is placed at risk (Rugg-Gunn et al., 1988).

Water fluoridation materially reduces the geographical differences in caries levels noted in the rest of the country and benefits mostly those children from deprived backgrounds, reducing the differences otherwise apparent between these children and those from more affluent families. This benefit occurs regardless of dietary or dental health habits or the availability of dental services.

In some countries, fluoridated salt has been used instead of fluoridating the water supplies, and the World Health Organization (WHO) has supported community studies into the value of adding fluoride to milk (WHO, 1994).

Expert opinion holds the view that the considerable improvement in the dental health of children that has occurred over the last quarter of a century in communities with suboptimal levels of fluoride in the water supplies, is due largely to the introduction of toothpastes containing fluoride (Bratthall et al., 1996). Controlled clinical trials have demonstrated reductions from the use of fluoride toothpastes of about 30% in the increment of caries, but when used over a life time it would appear that their effect is far greater than this (Davies et al., 1995). An important observation is that the regional variations in the levels of dental caries across Britain are mirrored by the sales of fluoride toothpaste, suggesting that their use may play a part in these differences (Davies et al., 1995).

It is recommended that all dentate people should brush their teeth twice a day with a fluoride toothpaste (HEA, 1996). In order to minimise the risk of cosmetically unacceptable fluorosis, parents of children below the age of 7 years are advised to supervise their offspring during toothbrushing, and to use only a small pea-sized amount of paste (BSPD, 1996).

Fluoride supplements (drops and tablets) might also help those living in communities with suboptimal levels of fluoride in their water supplies who their dentists judge are at risk of caries (BDA et al., 1997).

It is important that the improvements in the dental health of children are maintained and enhanced so that these trends may continue into adulthood. Patterns of behaviour established in childhood can be expected to make a large contribution to determining levels of health and patterns of dental service use in later life (Pitts, 1997). Therefore, children are a very important group to target for both health promotion and preventative programmes.

13.5 SUMMARY AND CONCLUSIONS

Although there has been a considerable reduction in the prevalence of dental caries among children over the last quarter of a century, caries is still an important health problem. The prevalence of caries is still declining among adolescents, but the improvement has ceased in young children. Even in pre-school years, the north–south gradient in the UK in caries prevalence and the high levels of the disease among children from families suffering multiple deprivation, are as apparent as they are in adolescence.

Extrinsic sugars are the most important dietary factor in the aetiology of dental caries among children and adolescents, and should be confined to meals. In infancy, those children having a drink containing sugar in a feeding bottle, particularly at bedtime, suffer from a greater prevalence and severity of caries than those who do not or those who have milk alone.

The regular use of a fluoride toothpaste, particularly if supervised by a parent, offers considerable protection against a sugar challenge. Chronically ill and disadvantaged children suffer more from the consequences of dental infections than do their healthy peers.

Although tooth-tissue loss among children and adolescents does not yet appear to be a problem of public health significance, for those seriously affected it can be a disfiguring condition. The main aetiological factor is thought to be the excessive consumption of acidic drinks.

Fluoridation of water at the optimal level of 1 ppm is an essential factor in the control of caries among children. All children should brush their teeth twice a day with a toothpaste containing fluoride.

14

OLDER PEOPLE

14.1 INTRODUCTION

The elderly are an important population group, since in virtually all industrialised countries including the UK, there is a greater percentage of the population surviving into old age. It is estimated that at the present time 8.44 million people in the UK are aged over 65 years (15.1% of the population). This is projected to increase to 9.78 million by the year 2020 (17.4% of the population) (Anonymous, 1985). There will be a contemporaneous change in the oral health status of this population cohort. Data from the 1988 adult dental health survey shows that 67% of the population aged 65 years or more had no natural teeth (were edentate). However, Todd and Lader (1991) provided population projections based on data over a 20-year period that suggest that this figure would fall to approximately 18% by 2038. A reduction in edentulousness is occurring throughout the industrialised world and will have a profound impact on the oral health care needs and disease susceptibility of this age group.

14.2 AGE-ASSOCIATED CHANGE

Increasing age has an inevitable, intrinsic and irreversible effect on all tissues of the body that are also manifest in changes to the oral and facial tissues.

14.2.1 Oral soft tissues and salivary glands

With ageing there are changes in the submucosa including alteration in collagen structure and turnover and reduced elasticity of elastin, a reduction in masticatory muscle bulk (Newton *et al.*, 1993) and profound reductions in the numbers of secretory units in salivary glands (Scott, 1987). Despite the marked histological changes in salivary gland structure seen in older people, there is little effect on salivary flow rates from the major salivary glands in this population

group (Baum, 1986; Närhi *et al.*, 1992). This is thought to be due to a combination of adaptive capacity on the part of the gland and increased vagal neurological tone seen in older people which will increase secretory activity. Nevertheless, the salivary secretory reserve is perceived to be lower in older people. Any challenges to salivary competence, including gland destruction by disease or radiotherapy or the side effects of drugs (Walls, 1998; Sreebny and Swartz, 1997) are more likely to produce xerostomia in this age group. There are also some suggestions in the literature that minor salivary gland function is diminished with age (Smith *et al.*, 1992; Gandara *et al.*, 1985).

There is a clinical impression that the oral mucosae become thinned and more friable with increasing age, but there are few data to support this other than on the lateral border of the tongue, where there is reduced epithelial thickness and a reduction in the complexity of the rete peg apparatus (Scott *et al.*, 1983). These alterations mirror the profound changes seen in skin with epithelial atrophy, increase in carbohydrate level and keratinisation that occur with age (Shklar, 1966; Scott *et al.*, 1983). Oral manifestations may also result from systemic age related diseases, e.g. atherosclerosis, which is commoner in older people, and may produce oral changes by a diminution in the blood supply leading to mucosal atrophy (Scott and Baum, 1990).

14.2.2 Taste

There is controversy in the literature in relation to age associated changes in taste, particularly as change in taste perception may be associated with variations in nutrient intake (Chauhan *et al.*, 1987). In addition there are well documented changes in smell with age (Chauhan *et al.*, 1987). The relationships between ageing and taste vary with both the taste quality (sweet, salt, sour and bitter) and variations in the intensity of the taste stimulus (Weiffenbach, 1987). Nevertheless, there are associations between increasing age and an increase in the thresholds for detection of sweet (Moore *et al.*, 1982) and salt (Baker *et al.*, 1983; Grzegorczyk *et al.*, 1979; Stevens *et al.*, 1991). Furthermore, there is some evidence for greater confusion between salt and sour in older subjects (Stevens and Cain, 1993) although the effects of mixture suppression on those tasting does not appear to be influenced by age (Stevens *et al.*, 1991; Stevens and Cain, 1993).

14.2.3 Teeth

Age has an impact both on the teeth and their supporting structures. Morphological age changes that affect erupted teeth include tooth wear, deposition of secondary dentine and cementum and root dentine translucency. The enamel and dentine undergo a surface maturation process with time because of continuous de- and remineralisation of the tooth surface during function. Teeth exposed to acids, either from the diet or the metabolic products of glucose metabolism by dental plaque bacteria including *Streptococci mutans*, will experience some surface demineralisation. Once the oral pH rises above the critical level (about pH 5.4 for enamel and pH 5.8 for dentine), saliva has the capacity to remineralise such areas. During this process, ions other than calcium and phosphate become incorporated within the surface mineral. These ions include fluoride as well as other trace elements for example selenium and manganese. This process results in a surface that is less soluble and permeable than not previously orally exposed dentine or enamel, consequently it is more resistant to decay.

14.3 DENTAL STATUS OF OLDER PEOPLE

Older people have fewer teeth than the young and are more likely to be reliant on a prosthesis of some sort for function. A variable proportion of the adult population will have no natural teeth. The most recent data for the UK (Steele *et al.*, 1998) suggest a rate of edentulousness of 50% for the over 65-year-old population. The rates of edentulousness are greater in the north of England and Scotland, and for people from manual social backgrounds and for women (Steele *et al.*, 1996, 1998).

14.3.1 The dentate

Amongst those with natural teeth (the dentate), increasing age is associated with a reduction in the numbers of teeth present, the number of

functional pairs of teeth (teeth which oppose each other) and the numbers of pairs of opposing posterior teeth. One measure of a functional dentition that has been suggested is the proportion of people who have 20 or more natural teeth (this is one of the World Health Organisation oral health targets) (WHO, 1989). Currently the average dentate over 65-year-old in Great Britain would have about 15 teeth, with about 29% having 21 or more teeth. These figures fall to an average of 10 teeth, with only 5% having 21 or more teeth for the over 85-year-olds. In addition, about 26% of dentate subjects over 65 years have no teeth in one dental arch with a complete denture in one jaw being opposed by natural teeth in the other. This last pattern of dental health seems to be particularly limiting in relation to food choice and, thus, nutrient intake (Steele *et al.*, 1998).

The crowns of teeth (the surfaces covered by dental enamel) are susceptible to decay throughout the life of the tooth from its eruption (between the ages of 6–18 years) to extraction or death. Conversely, the roots of teeth become exposed with increasing frequency in older patients because of gingival recession, mainly through periodontal disease. This results in new surfaces being exposed in older patients that are susceptible to decay.

The current cohort of dentate older people belong to a generation who have had some extensive restorative dental care in their youth. The legacy of this is a large number of heavily filled teeth retained in their mouths. Consequently, it is difficult to assess decay activity on the crowns of teeth, as this tends to take the form of recurrent decay around existing restorations. The limited data available on decay of crowns of teeth in older subjects suggests an increasing frequency of decay with increasing age (Steele *et al.*, 1998; Ambjornsen, 1986; Heft *et al.*, 1987; Winn *et al.*, 1996). This apparent increase in decay activity with age may be due to increasing disease activity or to reduced dental attendance resulting in more decayed surfaces being apparent during epidemiological studies of oral health for this age group.

Conversely, root decay has been more extensively studied, as it is of increased relevance in older people. Prevalence rates of between 60–90% have been demonstrated for older population groups (Galan and Lynch, 1993). The susceptible sites (the root surfaces of teeth) are exposed almost universally with increased age and hence there is greater risk of decay activity. Risk factors for active root decay include reduced salivary flow, increased age, gender and frequency of intake of sugars. Active decay is a condition concentrated within a small proportion of the population (80% of decayed lesions are present in about 20% of the population (Steele *et al.*, 1996)). Again, the older the subject, the more likely they are to have experienced root decay and to have untreated root decay in their mouths.

The signs of periodontal destruction are more severe in older people (Löe *et al.*, 1978; Carlos, 1987; Todd and Lader, 1991). This includes marked gingival recession in some patients in the absence of overt disease (Scott and Baum, 1990).

The pattern of periodontal destruction seen in older people appears to be different from the young. Shallow periodontal pockets are less likely to progress and deep pockets more likely to progress in an older age cohort. This is probably a consequence of two factors. First, a survivor effect in that those people who have teeth when they are 65 years old are unlikely to be amongst the groups most susceptible to periodontal breakdown. Second, there are alterations in the immune response with age which modify the pattern of disease activity (Holm-Pedersen *et al.*, 1975; Grbic and Lamster, 1991; Grbic and Lamster, 1992).

14.3.2 Masticatory function

As a broad generalisation, there is a decline in chewing ability with the reduction in the number functional pairs of natural teeth. The impact of this reduction is limited when there are 21 or more teeth remaining, corresponding to the shortened dental arch (Oosterhaven *et al.*, 1988; Carlos and Wolfe, 1989). However, where there are fewer than 21 teeth present there is a need to rely increasingly on a partial denture as an adjunct to function (Steele *et al.*, 1997), and objectively measured masticatory efficiency is reduced with or without the use of partial dentures (Gunne, 1985).

Masticatory efficiency with dentures is poorer than that with natural teeth. The least effective combination, from a masticatory standpoint, appears to be natural dentition in one jaw opposed by a complete denture in the opposing jaw.

14.4 ORAL HEALTH AND NUTRITION

A logical extension of the previous discussion on masticatory efficiency would be that reduced chewing ability would influence nutritional status. This area of work has been somewhat neglected, however, there are some data avail-

able, most recently from the National Diet and Nutrition Survey for people aged 65 years and over in Great Britain (Steele *et al.*, 1998). A comparable study has also been conducted in the USA (Kleinman and Drury, 1996); unfortunately, as yet, no analysis of the relationships between oral health and nutritional status have been conducted on these data. Farrell (1956, 1957) established some time ago that chewing was not necessarily required for digestion of a modern diet. However, inefficient masticatory ability influences food choice which in turn has an effect on both intake and nutritional status in older subjects. People with reduced masticatory efficiency are less able to eat foods that require rigourous chewing, for example apples, raw carrots, nuts, toast, tomatoes, crisps and oranges. This observation is valid both for those with reduced numbers of teeth in the natural dentition, and for those who are edentate (Carlos and Wolfe, 1989; Steele *et al.*, 1998).

These variations in ability to eat food are also reflected in variations in nutrient intake in relation to intrinsic and milk sugars and non-starch polysaccharide for dentate subjects. The greater the numbers of pairs of occluding teeth and of pairs of posterior occluding teeth present in older people, the more intrinsic and milk sugars and non-starch polysaccharides they consume (Österberg and Steen, 1982; Steele *et al.*, 1998). Protein, intrinsic and milk sugars, calcium, non-haem iron, niacin and vitamin C intake are also consumed in greater amounts in the dentate compared with the edentate (Heath, 1971; Moynihan *et al.*, 1994; Steele *et al.*, 1998).

Finally, haematological and biochemical measures of nutritional status are also influenced by oral health status. Plasma ascorbate (vitamin C) is lower in edentate subjects and in those with fewer pairs of opposing teeth. Plasma retinol (vitamin A) and α-tocopherol (vitamin E) levels were also reduced in edentate subjects compared with the dentate (Steele *et al.*, 1998).

The impact of these nutritional deficiencies is unclear. It is worth noting that in addition to the above data, some of the subgroups within the National Diet and Nutrition Survey had particularly poor nutritional status for specific micronutrients. For example the median plasma ascorbate level for edentate subjects living in an institution was 11.4 μmol/l, at the extreme lower range of normal. By definition, 50% of this sample would have plasma ascorbate levels lower than this value. This is of particular concern when the associations between vitamin C status and respiratory function, and the risks of stroke and cardiovascular disease are taken into consideration (Khaw and Woodhouse, 1995; Ness *et al.*, 1996a, b, c).

14.5 NUTRITION AND ORAL HEALTH

There is an increased prevalence of exposure of the roots of the teeth in older people to the oral environment. The exposed dentine is susceptible to decay, with many factors contributing towards the aetiology of decay in this group. One of the factors is the frequency of ingestion of sugars (Steele *et al.*, 1998; Papas *et al.*, 1995).

People who have a dry mouth, either as a result of pathological changes in the glands or of pharmacological suppression of salivary output, have particular difficulties, and efforts must be made to stimulate their salivary flow. A common problem is that people use strong gustatory stimuli to improve salivary activity often in the form of strong peppermint or menthol flavoured sweets. These items can have a high sugar content which, if used frequently in a patient with reduced salivary buffering capacity and flow rate, will result in rapidly progressing decay on multiple vulnerable surfaces. Furthermore, acid-containing stimuli should be avoided to reduce the risk of both root decay and tooth wear in this population group (Walls, 1998).

Excessive consumption of foods and beverages containing dietary acids should also be avoided in those identified as at risk of an erosive pattern of tooth wear (Järvinnen *et al.*, 1991).

Nutritional deficiency states in older people may result in alterations in oral mucosal integrity, exacerbating the age-associated changes in the structure of this tissue. The micronutrients most commonly associated with mucosal pathology include iron, vitamin B_{12} and folate. In addition to their effects on oral mucosa, such deficiency is also associated with *Candida albicans* infection at the angles of the mouth (*angular cheilitis*) (Scully, 1989). Such deficiency states are more prevalent in older population groups (Morley, 1986).

14.6 SUMMARY AND CONCLUSIONS

Significant oral changes are associated with ageing, both because of ageing itself and a lifetime's function of the dentition in the oral environment. These changes result in an oral cavity whose mucosa is likely to be more susceptible to damage because of nutritional deficiencies should they occur.

The reduction in numbers of pairs of functional teeth in the dentate and the reduced effectiveness of dentures in the edentate result in altered foods choice; this in turn leads to some alterations in nutrient intake and nutritional status of subjects. Some of these effects contribute to levels of nutritional status that are close to deficiency states and are likely to have an effect on the overall health and welfare of the individual.

15

PEOPLE LIVING IN AREAS OF MULTIPLE DEPRIVATION

15.1 MEASURES OF DEPRIVATION

The evidence that social and economic variations exist and impact on oral health and related behaviours is substantial. Several methods have been used in dental research to classify people according to their social class or socioeconomic status. The most popular method is to use the Registrar General's classification of the occupation of the head of the household (OPCS, 1980). However, this has come under increasing criticism particularly as a significant proportion of society are now included in the 'Unclassified' category. More recently, a number of deprivation indexes have been developed to assign residents within a geographical area with a relative deprivation score, e.g. the ACORN classification of residential neighbourhoods, the Townsend material deprivation score and the Jarman index. All depend to a certain extent on the material resources available and therefore consider not only individual circumstances, but also the wider community and environmental issues which affect individual lifestyles. Therefore, quantifying multiple deprivation is complex and embraces a wide range of factors from poor environmental conditions, cultural and racial disadvantage, to low income levels. Individuals may experience only one of these, but it is the cumulative effect of multiple deprivation that significantly affects health.

15.2 ORAL HEALTH AND DEPRIVATION

The national surveys of child (O'Brien, 1994) and adult dental health (Todd and Lader, 1991) have established that the levels of oral diseases and their treatment are worse in people from the manual classes than in those from the non-manual classes. This is clearly apparent in children, where most of the dental caries is now found in a reducing proportion of the population who are heavily orientated towards the deprived families, and in the elderly where edentulousness is concentrated in working class people.

Several studies have demonstrated that the prevalence of caries in pre-school children of materially disadvantaged families is higher than in those of wealthier families (Sutcliffe, 1977; Holt et al., 1988). It has also been shown that the children of poorer families have an increased frequency of intake of sugar-containing foods and beverages, and have their teeth brushed less often with fluoride toothpaste (Jones et al., 1996). This was also demonstrated in the National Diet and Nutrition Survey of infants and young children (Hinds and Gregory, 1995). The factors associated with this were the use of infant feeding bottles, dinky feeders and dummies, the consumption of sugary drinks at bedtime and the consumption of confectionery and carbonated beverages (Hinds and Gregory, 1995). A lower level of caries occurred in those who consumed confectionery and carbonated drinks infrequently and who brushed their teeth most often. Frequent brushing did not fully counteract the detrimental effect of frequent sugar consumption. However, in multiple regression analysis socioeconomic factors were important (Moyniham and Holt, 1996; Hinds and Gregory, 1995).

A study of the dental health of pre-school children in Norway (Grytten et al., 1988) used the educational level of the mother as an indicator of social class. Once again, the children of mothers with less formal education had the higher level of caries, the most unfavourable behaviour in relation to caries being frequent sugar consumption. Blinkhorn (1982) showed the same relationship in a study conducted in Edinburgh, agreeing with a similar, earlier conclusion from research in the same city (Sutcliffe, 1977).

The inverse relationship of caries prevalence with social class has also been established in children of school age (Carmichael et al., 1980; Bradnock et al., 1984; O'Brien, 1994). Bradnock *et al.* (1984) showed the influence of social class on caries experience to be stronger than that of water fluoridation, although fluoridation does considerably reduce the absolute difference between the social classes (Evans *et al.*, 1996).

The National Adult Dental Health Survey (Todd and Lader, 1991) showed that people from unskilled, manual households were more likely to be edentulous than those from other social classes. Among those who possessed teeth, working class adults had fewer teeth on average than adults from middle class households. They were also more likely to have untreated, decayed teeth, and less likely to have diseased teeth filled. Adults from manual, unskilled backgrounds were also likely to have worse periodontal health. Adults from social classes IV and V were more likely to attend the dentist only when they had trouble with their teeth, were more fearful of attending, and wanted an aching tooth extracted rather than filled. They were also less likely to take time off from work to attend for dental treatment.

15.3 NUTRITION, ORAL HEALTH AND DEPRIVATION

The simple answer to poorer oral health among those living in areas of multiple deprivation might be to exhort these communities to eat a more healthy diet, breast-feed their babies, stop giving their infants sugary drinks from feeding bottles, stop their children eating confectionery frequently, clean their teeth twice a day using a fluoride toothpaste and visit a dentist regularly. In fact, much of our formal dental health education does just that, however, some people appreciate that it is not that simple. Poverty restricts freedom of choice almost as much as illness. Poverty has a dramatic influence upon an individual's and a family's diet. It affects their choice and selection of food, as well as their purchasing patterns. A recent study exploring dietary choice among disadvantaged groups indicated that parents went without food in order that their children were able to enjoy 'treats' such as confectionery and biscuits (Dowler and Calvert, 1993). Bennett *et al.* (1995) found a clear relationship between social class and reported use of sugar. For example, men in social classes IV and V were more likely to say that they added sugar to tea (60%) than those in social classes I and II (36%). Among women, 47% of those in social classes IV and V said they added sugar to coffee compared with 27% of those in social classes I and II.

Dowler and Calvert (1995) found that lone-par-

ents on low incomes prioritised their needs, made do, or did without. This has been confirmed in a Family Policy and Parenthood Practice Survey which showed that low-income families developed strategies for coping and managing their budgets in the short-term, but were unlikely to do any long-term planning with regard to diet (Dobson *et al.*, 1994). These difficulties are compounded by the relatively poor selection of fresh foodstuffs that is available within many inner city environments (Dowler and Calvert, 1995).

These behaviours will have dramatic effects upon oral health. A study comparing the dental health of primary school children from different social groups within a single community (Gratrix and Holloway, 1994) suggested that materially-deprived parents were able to exercise so little control over their lives, and those of their children, that they were unable to socialise them to acceptable behaviour. The groups with the higher caries experience had higher Townsend mean deprivation scores, lower percentages of private housing, fewer households with a car, and were reported to have a higher proportion of financial and social problems. More of the children received clothing allowances and free school meals. The high caries groups had lower proportions of babies of normal birth weight and there were lower uptakes of poliomyelitis vaccination in children born to single parent families. The mothers in these groups tended to bottle-feed their babies, wean them earlier, use infant feeding bottles longer and give their babies juice drinks more regularly. Their children had poorer attendance and punctuality records at infant school, were worse behaved and had more sweets after school.

The association between diet and poverty is well accepted. The adverse impact of poverty, diet and general health in the UK continues to cause debate. However, significant variations in oral health exist among different socioeconomic groups and strong evidence from the literature shows that deprived communities consume more cariogenic foodstuffs and their eating patterns are more likely to give rise to dental caries (Bennett *et al.*, 1993; Dowler and Calvert, 1995).

The annual Food Survey of 7000 British households shows that, compared with the highest income group, low income groups consume more milk (but less semi-skimmed milk), meat and meat products (especially higher fat meat products), fats, sugar and preserves, potatoes and cereals (MAFF 1995, 1996; James *et al.*, 1997).

Parents with limited resources cannot afford

to discard food that their children refuse. This means that they must purchase foods that are acceptable to their families rather than the food that nutritionists recommend (Dobson *et al.*, 1994). In families with children, expenditure on food per person in the bottom fifth of income level is low (£1.64/person/day in lone parent families) (Central Statistical Office, 1996). However, low socioeconomic groups allocate a greater proportion of their income to food, and purchase more food per unit of expenditure than high income households. This means that they buy food that is high in fat and sugar to ensure that their children receive sufficient calories (Central Statistical Office, 1996; James *et al.*, 1997).

In addition to appropriate health education, food manufacturers should apply their technology to increasing the choice and availability of inexpensive foods that are attractive to children yet are low in fat and sugar and high in complex carbohydrates and fibre. These need to be advertised attractively to them.

15.4 SUMMARY AND CONCLUSIONS

There is clear evidence that social and economic inequalities impact upon oral health and eating patterns. Poverty restricts choice in food purchasing and low income families are more likely to consume a more cariogenic diet and have a poor dental attendance pattern. Further research is required into effective oral health promotion strategies among 'at risk' population groups, and special resources should be made available to improve the access to treatment for children from such communities.

16

CULTURE AND DIET

16.1 INTRODUCTION

Dietary and lifestyle information for minority ethnic groups is limited, and only recently has information been gathered on a national basis (Pacy, 1989; Rudat, 1994). The 1997 National Infant-feeding Survey in Asian families is the most comprehensive information on ethnic variations in breast-feeding and weaning patterns to date (Thomas and Avery, 1997).

In considering the influence of culture and diet on health in the UK's minority ethnic groups, it is important to highlight that food habits are primarily associated with four variables; ethnic and historical background, religious affiliation, the degree of acculturation to 'British culture' and socioeconomic status.

16.2 ETHNIC AND HISTORICAL BACKGROUND

The 1991 Census of Population have included for the first time, a question on the ethnic group of respondents (Table 16.1). This made it possible for the size and type of minority ethnic communities to be assessed (Owen, 1996). The great advantage of the ethnic information derived from the census is that it helps remove the previous reliance on country of birth as a proxy for ethnicity (Coleman and Salt, 1996).

The minority ethnic population in England and Wales is currently estimated to be 6% of the total population (Table 16.2). The minority ethnic groups are not evenly distributed, but clustered in different localities. These tend to be urban (Owen, 1996), with less than 1% living in rural areas. At the extreme, Greater London contains 12.2% of the total population of Great Britain, but nearly half (45%) of Britain's minority ethnic population (Storkey and Lewis, 1996).

The largest single minority ethnic group is Indian, which forms 1.5% of the whole UK population, and 28% of the minority ethnic population (Owen, 1996). The second largest is the Black Caribbean group, which constitutes 17% of the latter. The introduction of the ethnic question in the census was innovative, but in the final analysis there was a simplification of the ethnic categories by merging some categories into single groups (e.g. Punjabis, Gujaratis and Tamils were all covered by the one term 'Indian') (Table 16.1).

The age structure of the minority ethnic population differs from that of the indigenous group, such that in the former there is a greater proportion of younger individuals (Warnes, 1996). Three in five people from minority ethnic groups are under the age of 30 years, compared with two in five of the population as a whole. In the Bangladeshi, Pakistani and 'Black other' groups, about half are under the age of 16 years (Owen,1996).

An understanding of traditional diet in countries from which migration has taken place, may provide some insight into present eating habits. However, the diversity between groups make generalisation of dietary customs difficult (Pacy, 1989). Diets of Gujarati women living in Harrow, England, have a higher fat and lower carbohydrate and fibre content than those of women living in Gujarat, India (Abrahams, 1983). The sample of women included also had a higher intake of sucrose and refined cereals than their contemporaries in Gujarat (Abrahams, 1983).

The National Survey of Infant-feeding in Asian families showed some ethnic variations in breast-feeding and weaning patterns (Thomas and Avery, 1997). The incidence of breast-feeding was 90% among Bangladeshi, 82% among Indian, 76% among Pakistani and 62% among White mothers. However, of mothers who started to breast feed, Pakistani and Bangladeshi women stopped breast-feeding sooner than either Indian or White women. Bangladeshi mothers were the most concerned about having sufficient milk, and one in five gave this as a reason for planning to give a bottle as well as breast feed (Thomas and Avery, 1997). It was also the Bangladeshi mothers who were the most likely to add sugar to the milk in their baby's bottle. By 15 months, both Bangladeshi and Pakistani mothers were more likely to add rusks and sugar to their baby's bottle compared

Table 16.1 The 1991 Census of Population ethnic classification

Four-group classification	Ten-group classification	Full listing
White	White	White Irish Greek/Greek Cypriot Turkish/Turkish Cypriot Mixed White
Black groups	Black: Caribbean	Black: Caribbean Caribbean Island West Indies Guyana
	Black: African	Black: African African south of the Sahara
	Black: Other	Black: other Black: British Black: Mixed Black/White Black: Mixed other
Indian/Pakistani/Bangladeshi	Indian Pakistani Bangladeshi	Indian Pakistani Bangladeshi
Chinese and others	Chinese	Chinese
	Other: Asian	East African Asian Indo-Caribbean Black: Indian subcontinent Black: other Asian
	Other: Other	North African/Arab/Iranian Mixed Asian/White British ethnic minority (other) British (no indication) Other mixed Black/White Other mixed Asian/White Other mixed-Other

Source: Ratcliffe (1996). © Crown Copyright. Reproduced with permission: Office for National Statistics.

to other groups (Thomas and Avery, 1997). The effects of this behaviour are reflected in epidemiological evidence of higher levels of dental caries among young children from these two ethnic groups compared to non-Muslim Asian groups and White children (Bedi and Elton, 1991).

The concerns of health professionals with regard to diet have been centred primarily on nutritional deficiencies of iron and of vitamins B_{12} and D in certain Asian populations, betel quid and tobacco chewing, and the custom of including ghee (clarified butter) in cooking. Other concerns have been about the changes in eating habits of second generation minority ethnic groups. A study investigating changes in diet and oral health related behaviours between inner city first and second generation Pakistani

mothers resident in the UK, showed that for this group negative health attitudes were resistant to change (Godson et al., 1996). Infant-feeding practices had not altered in the succeeding generation, but the frequency of intake of cariogenic foods had, with second generation mothers giving their children higher levels of sucrose-containing foods (Godson et al., 1996). Other concerns related to health have centred on the use of lead-based cosmetics (surma) (Smaje, 1995).

16.3 RELIGIOUS AFFILIATION

Religious affiliation may play a major role in determining dietary practices. Traditional beliefs about diet and health, religious restrictions and

Table 16.2 Population change in ethnic minority groups in Great Britain (1981–91)

Group	Population 1981 (000s)	Population 1991 (000s)	Change 1981–91 (000s)	% change 1981–91
White	52,600.0	53,062.3	452.3	0.9
Black: Caribbean	422.5	522.2	99.7	23.6
Black: African	141.4	219.2	77.8	55.0
Black: Other	143.8	188.2	44.5	30.9
Black groups	707.7	929.6	21.9	31.4
Indian	627.8	877	249.2	39.7
Pakistani	344.5	500.3	155.8	45.2
Bangladeshi	87.8	171.5	83.8	95.4
South Asian groups	1,060.1	1,548.8	488.8	46.1
Chinese	11.5	160.8	49.3	44.2
Other: Asian	110.4	202.3	91.9	83.2
Other: Other	214	302.2	88.2	41.2
Other: Groups	435.9	665.3	229.4	52.6
All ethnic minorities	2,203.7	3,143.7	940.1	42.7
Total	54,813	56,206.1	1,392.4	2.5

Source: Rees and Phillips (1996). © Crown Copyright. Reproduced with permission: Office for National Statistics.

patterns of abstaining from food affect food choice as well as times of consumption. This is also true for tobacco and alcohol use.

In the UK there are six sizeable faith communities: Buddhism, Christianity, Hinduism, Islam, Judaism and Sikhism.

There are a number of Buddhist sects, but the two main schools are Mahayana, prevalent in China and Japan, and Therevada, prevalent in South-East Asia. Some Buddhists abstain from eating on the first and fifteenth day of each lunar month, but there are no other specific dietary regulations within the religion.

Christianity is the largest faith community in the UK. Amongst minority ethnic communities, Christianity attracts predominantly those of Black Caribbean origin. There are few, if any, specific dietary restrictions within the Christian religion.

Hinduism is widespread among the Asian community, especially amongst those from India and East Africa. Regular fasting can form part of religious practice but this varies between denominations. The majority of Hindus do not eat meat or fish. Alcohol is officially disapproved of, but not forbidden.

Muslim are followers of the Islamic faith. Most Muslims in the UK are from Pakistan and Bangladesh. Eating pork in any form is forbidden in Islam. Other meat may be eaten, provided it is *halal* (killed in the manner prescribed by Islamic

law). Alcohol is strictly prohibited. Muslims are required to fast from dawn to dusk during the holy month of Ramadan.

The Jewish community in Britain is diverse and religious dietary regulations vary. Pork and its derivatives and shellfish are strictly prohibited by Jewish law. All other meat or meat derived products should be *kosher* which requires that it has been slaughtered according to Jewish law.

The Sikh community is closely linked with North West India and parts of Pakistan. Meat is not specifically prohibited but many Sikhs avoid eating pork.

The major areas of investigation with regard to diet and religious affiliation have been in relation to the South Asian and, particularly, the Islamic community. Levels of breast-feeding by South Asian mothers are lower than amongst their indigenous counterparts (Aukett and Wharton, 1989). In addition there are noticeable differences in health related behaviours in Islamic households, in that Muslim men often carry out the majority of food shopping (Wharton and Wharton, 1989). This is less true in Hindu and Sikh households. Although similar levels of carbohydrate intake are seen in Pakistani Muslims, Sikhs and Hindus, it is noticeable that this is higher in the Bangladeshi Muslim group (Wharton and Wharton, 1989).

16.4   ACCULTURATION

Several definitions have been used to describe culture. Leniniger (1988) defined culture in a society as the 'learned, shared and transmitted values, beliefs, norms and life practices of a particular group'. Therefore, culture is dynamic, flexible, variable and adaptable. Changes in culture are displayed in patterns of, and responses to, health and illness (Kiyak, 1993). Culture includes the transmission of norms or patterned beliefs and behaviours that often determine interpretations of disease symptoms and aetiology, health seeking behaviours and acceptability of treatment regimens.

Suchman and Rothman (1993) compared ethnic groups on three aspects of health care and responses to illness, and classified ethnic groups into 'parochial' (ethnocentric, traditional, closed social groups) or 'cosmopolitan' (open, progressive, individualistic). Although simplistic, this binary subgrouping gives expression to the dynamic nature of culture as being not a single entity, but having many subcultures within it. These subcultures express themselves in their interaction within the main host culture and in their traditional cultural heritage. This inter-reaction process is referred to as 'acculturation'.

Acculturation refers to a complex process whereby a minority group—as a result of its continuous exposure to a cultural system that is significantly different from its own—modifies its social norms, attitudes, values and behaviours, relinquishing some characteristics of the culture of origin (Ramirez, 1980).

The acculturation process is significantly influenced by ethnic and historical background, religious affiliation and socioeconomic status. Migrants from the Caribbean and Africa entered the UK with few linguistic problems compared to the South Asian and Chinese communities. In addition, their dietary patterns and religious affiliations made the process of acculturation easier than for the latter two groups. For the Islamic populations in particular, their religious restrictions act as major barriers to developing the acculturation process. However, age is also significantly linked with acculturation. Currently, over half of the Bangladeshi (Muslim) community are under 16 years of age. These individuals were born in the UK, and their process of acculturation is likely to be more developed than amongst older groups (Owen, 1996; Warnes, 1996).

No studies have reported directly on oral health status or on behaviour and acculturation levels of minority ethnic groups in the UK. How-ever, in the USA, Ismail et al. (1990) showed Mexican-Americans with lower acculturation levels had a higher mean number of decayed and missing teeth, compared to those with high levels of acculturation. Spolsky et al. (1996) also found the dental caries experience in a Hispanic sample from Los Angeles was significantly related to the level of acculturation, with those who had not adapted so well having higher levels of caries. However, the measurement of acculturation was simply based on the ability to speak English. Socioeconomic status variables are strongly related to the process of acculturation, especially educational background, employment status and occupation.

16.5   SOCIOECONOMIC STATUS

Food choice in the minority ethnic groups is determined not only by tradition, knowledge and experience, but also by social and economic factors affecting the availability and affordability of foods.

There is strong evidence that in the UK, as in most industrialised countries, minority ethnic groups are disadvantaged in many aspects of social and economic life (Pearson, 1991; Brown, 1984). Groups which are distinctive either due to their skin colour, facial features or cultural behaviour have tended to occupy low social positions, and are subject to discrimination which serves to maintain their disadvantaged status.

Given that both socioeconomic status and ethnicity variables are frequently ill defined, due to the amalgamation of diverse and complex groupings which conceal major intragroup differences, the potential for residual confounding is high. Few studies have attempted to quantify the combined effects of poverty and ethnic discrimination, or what Spencer (1996) refers to as the 'double jeopardy'.

The 1991 census showed that although a greater proportion of Black and Asian people in the UK have Higher-education Degrees than the White population, they are twice as likely to be unemployed. So far as the distribution of income is concerned, 40% of Indian and 50% of Pakistani and Bangladeshi Britons are found in the bottom 20%. These factors have direct health outcomes, for example, births to Pakistani mothers in the UK have persistently higher rates of perinatal mortality and lower birthweights (Pearson, 1991). The latter will have significant influence on both dental caries risk and levels of enamel defects.

17

ILL-HEALTH AND DISEASE

The integrity of the oral tissues relies on an adequate supply of nutrients and elements, which in turn are supplied by a balanced diet. Ill-health or disease, however, can compromise this nutrient supply in a number of different ways. Adequacy of the diet is dependent on a plentiful food supply, and on the ability of the individual to consume appropriate amounts and types of foods. Individuals with diminished intellectual capacity, e.g. those suffering dementia or psychiatric disease, may be prone to nutritionally induced disease. Patients with physical handicap may also be unable, without help, to prepare or eat an adequate diet. Thus, those with cerebral palsy, Parkinsonism, arthritis or amputation may be malnourished and develop consequent poor oral health. Both diet and oral health can be inadequate due to general disability in ill-health, and hospitalised patients may, through neglect or lack of opportunity, have reduced oral hygiene and an impoverished diet leading to oral and dental disease.

The gastro-intestinal tract is the site of the absorption of food, and gastro-intestinal disease may lead to malnutrition through malabsorption or due to blood or nutrient loss from the gastro-intestinal tract. Malabsorption states include coeliac disease (gluten sensitive enteropathy), which arises due to atrophy of the intestinal villi caused by the α-gliadin component of cereal products in sensitive individuals. This in turn causes deficiencies of iron, folate and vitamin B_{12} and associated fat malabsorption. Other malabsorptive states include Crohn's disease and cystic fibrosis. The former is an inflammatory bowel disease which causes malabsorption, particularly of vitamin B_{12}, due to regional ileitis and iron deficiency due to gastro-intestinal blood loss. Cystic fibrosis causes malabsorption, particularly of fat, as a result of a lack of pancreatic enzymes. Finally, gut amyloid causes folate malabsorption and is seen in patients with rheumatoid arthritis who also have iron deficiency anaemia due to lack of iron utilisation, but who have normal iron stores.

The surgical removal of segments of the bowel can lead to decreased absorption, and gastrectomy can cause vitamin B_{12} deficiency due to removal of the cells that produce intrinsic factor. Diarrhoea may lead to loss of proteins, and gastro-intestinal blood loss due to haemorrhoids, peptic ulceration or bowel cancer can lead to iron deficiency anaemia.

The most frequent cause of iron deficiency anaemia in women in the UK is heavy menstrual blood loss, and about 20% of women in England aged between 18 and 54 years of age can be considered to have low iron stores (White *et al.*, 1993). Thus, anaemia is quite common and concomitant deficiencies may compromise oral health. Other causes of nutrient loss, rather than blood loss, include renal dialysis, and patients on regular dialysis may become deficient in trace elements such as zinc or magnesium. Nutrient loss due to exfoliation is rare, but patients with erythroderma due to psoriasis become folate deficient. Patients on tube or parenteral feeding may be susceptible to vitamin and mineral deficiencies with the resultant oral diseases described elsewhere.

Finally, drug therapy may compromise nutritional status by antagonising enzyme pathways such as with aminopterin, a cytotoxic drug that works by folate antagonism and, thus, can cause oral mucosal ulceration. Drug therapy may also compromise nutritional status by competing for absorption pathways, e.g. folate deficiency caused by phenytoin for epilepsy, or by inducing blood loss within the gastro-intestinal tract, e.g. with non-steroidal anti-inflammatories causing gastric bleeding.

Table 17.1   Diseases affecting oral health

Condition	Effect	Reference
Cardiovascular disease	Digoxin induced vomiting	Royal Pharmaceutical Society of Great Britain
Hypertension (antihypertensives)	Xerostomia; sialosis; pain; gingival hyperplasia	Royal Pharmaceutical Society of Great Britain
Leukaemias	Mucosal ulceration due to folate deficiency	Wray and Dagg (1990)
Cystic fibrosis	Ulcers (induced by pancreatic enzyme replacement); caries (induced by low fat, high carbohydrate diet); bleeding due to vitamin K deficiency	Fernald et al. (1990) Kinirons (1989) Primosch (1980) Tynam and Kamiyama (1984)
Coeliac disease	Dental malformation	Cook and Holmes (1984) Ramussen and Espelia (1980)
Diabetes mellitis	Sialosis; drug induced lichenoid eruptions; gingivitis and periodontal disease	Gislen et al. (1980) Murrah (1985)
Rickets/osteomalacia	Delayed eruption of teeth; jaw radiolucency	Seow and Latham (1986)
Gastric reflux (acid regurgitation)	Dental erosion	Järvinen et al. (1988)
Bulimia nervosa	Dental erosion; sialosis; angular cheilitis	Abrams and Ruff (1986) Clark (1985) Walsh et al. (1981)

18

GENERAL CONCLUSIONS AND RECOMMENDATIONS

CONCLUSIONS

1 Dental caries

1.1 *Prevalence*

- There have been substantial reductions in dental caries in the UK population in the last quarter of a century, especially amongst children. These reductions are now reflected in the lower caries level in young adults.
- Nevertheless, the prevalence of dental caries in the UK remains at an unacceptable level and while not life threatening, it is still a serious public health issue, e.g. two-thirds of 15-year-olds go into adulthood with some evidence of previous or existing caries.
- The reduction in dental caries appears to have ceased in the very young, and the rate of decrease has slowed down in adolescents.
- The size of the reduction in dental caries has not been uniform across all sectors of the population, e.g. the level of caries in groups suffering multiple deprivation is much higher than in the rest of the population and this difference is increasing; caries in the North of the UK is more prevalent than in the South.

1.2 *Multifactorial aspects*

The causes of caries are multifactorial and include:

- the biological influences at the tooth surface, e.g. microorganisms, plaque, saliva, sugars and other dietary components, fluoride;
- behavioural factors, e.g. eating habits and oral hygiene practices;
- the environment, e.g. social, geographical, water supply.

1.3 *Effects of diet*

- Sugars are the most important dietary aetiological determinant of dental caries.
- The main dietary sugars which cause caries are those that are free in, and added to, foods and drinks (sometimes classified as *extrinsic sugars*). The added sugar currently consumed in the greatest quantities is sucrose.
- There is no epidemiological evidence to demonstrate that sugars that are enclosed in the cellular structure of food (sometimes classified as *intrinsic sugars*) have an important influence on the development of dental caries, in the current patterns of dietary intake in the UK.
- The frequency and amount of sugars consumed are related, i.e. a greater frequency of intake of sugars is usually associated with a greater total intake.
- The frequency, duration and amount of consumption of sugar-containing foods and drinks are related to dental caries. The length of time sugars remain in contact with tooth surfaces is particularly important.
- There is no epidemiological evidence to demonstrate that the consumption of foods that are rich in starch without the addition of sugars, in the current patterns of dietary intake in the UK, plays a significant part in the aetiology of dental caries.
- Normally milk plays no part in the aetiology of dental caries, and may have a slight protective function.
- In the UK and other industrialised nations, the nutritional status of individuals (fluoride apart) has little influence on their resistance to dental caries.

1.4 *Effects of fluoride*

- Fluoride is the most important prophylactic agent against dental caries.

Optimal exposure to fluoride can halve the occurrence of dental caries.

- The decline in dental caries in the UK over the last quarter of a century can be attributed mainly to the regular use of fluoride toothpaste.
- Water fluoridation is the best researched and documented of all public health measures, and one of the most effective. It has been carried out in some areas of the UK for more than 40 years.
- The safety of water fluoridation at optimum levels has been pronounced by many authoritative scientific bodies in the UK and elsewhere, and has been further corroborated by several exhaustive examinations of the scientific evidence in courts of law.
- The beneficial influence of water fluoridation counteracts, to some extent, the geographical and social variations in dental caries.
- The main protective action of fluoride delivered by any method, including water fluoridation, is topical, i.e. it acts on the erupted tooth surface, rather than during tooth development.
- The most important factor in fluoride's effect in controlling dental caries, irrespective of the method of delivery, is the maintenance of an optimal level at the tooth surface.
- Some concerns have been expressed about the effect of excessive fluoride intake on health. These concerns have not been substantiated by an acceptable body of evidence.

2 Periodontal diseases

- Periodontal disease, at a level severe enough to risk the loss of some teeth, affects about one-sixth of the adult population in the UK.
- In the UK and other industrialised nations, diet and nutritional status have little effect on periodontal diseases (including gingivitis). Gingivitis is readily reversed by adequate oral hygiene.

3 Oral cancer

- In the UK, oral cancer represents 1–2% of total cancer incidence. Its occurrence appears to be increasing, especially in males under the age of 64 years, and

the age of presentation appears to be decreasing.

- Tobacco and alcohol are the main independent risk factors. Their combined use has a very strong adverse effect.
- South Asian immigrant communities in the UK have a high use of chewing tobacco, which may place them at an increased risk of oral cancer.
- Epidemiological studies indicate that high fruit and vegetable consumption may have a protective effect.

4 Tooth defects

4.1 Dental fluorosis

- The diagnosis of fluorosis is infrequent and uncertain. Cosmetically unacceptable fluorosis is infrequent in relation to the overwhelming numbers who benefit from fluoride in the control of dental caries.
- Water fluoridated at the level of 1 ppm (1 mg/l) may result in a slight increase in the number of individuals with very mild fluorosis; fluoride ingested from foods is not implicated in the development of cosmetically unacceptable fluorosis.
- There is no established evidence linking fluorosis to the appropriate use of fluoride toothpaste.

4.2 Enamel hypoplasia

- In the UK and other industrialised nations, diet and nutritional status after birth play little or no part in enamel hypoplasia. Maternal vitamin D deficiency during pregnancy has been associated with enamel hypoplasia in the infant.

4.3 Tooth-tissue loss

- Non-carious tooth-tissue loss includes erosion, abrasion and attrition and most often results from a combination of these.
- National population prevalence data of non-carious tooth-tissue loss are limited to two dental surveys of children and one of older people. Population data in other age groups are lacking.
- Acidic foods and drinks have the potential to erode tooth surfaces.

RECOMMENDATIONS

The Task Force proposes that the following recommendations should be made:

1 Recommendations to individuals

1.1 *Dental caries*

- Brush teeth twice a day with a fluoride toothpaste of proven efficacy; fluoride toothpaste will help prevent dental caries and the action of toothbrushing may help to control periodontal diseases.
- Limit the consumption of sugary foods and drinks to mealtimes.
- Avoid cariogenic snacks, and avoid cariogenic drinks including tea and coffee with added sugar, between meals.
- When feeding infants:
  - Do not add sugars to a bottle of infant formula or follow-on formula.
  - Do not allow babies with teeth to fall asleep while breast- or bottle-feeding.
  - Do not give fruit juices or other drinks containing sugars or other fermentable carbohydrate in bottles or reservoir feeders, especially at bedtime.
  - Ensure as far as possible that medicines given to infants and children are sugar-free.

1.2 *Oral cancer*

- Avoid the habit of tobacco use, including smoking and chewing.
- Limit alcohol consumption. Current recommendations for maximum daily intakes are between three and four units for men, and two and three units for women.
- Consume a balanced diet including a high intake of fruit and vegetables. Current recommendations are for five portions of different fruit and vegetables per day.
- Seek professional advice if experiencing a sore spot or ulcer in the mouth which lasts for more than three weeks.

1.3 *Tooth defects*

- Ensure that children under seven years of age use only a small pea-sized amount of fluoride toothpaste twice a day, are supervised by a responsible person while brushing their teeth, and are en-

couraged to spit out the paste, to avoid cosmetically unacceptable fluorosis.
- Use fluoride tablets and drops only on the advice of a dentist.

2 Recommendations to Health Authorities

- Endeavour to persuade water companies to fluoridate public water supplies.
- Collect more explanatory data on groups known to be at higher risk of dental caries, oral cancer and other oral diseases.
- Target oral health promotion at these 'at risk' groups.
- Provide ongoing training of all health professionals to ensure consistency of messages in the promotion of oral health (refer to *Recommendations to individuals* above), and make available specific training in cross-cultural counselling where necessary.

3 Recommendations to Local Government

- Support the work and efforts of Health Authorities in the promotion of oral health.
- Enforce existing national legislation restricting the advertising, sale and consumption of tobacco and alcohol products more effectively.

4 Recommendations to Central Government

- Amend the Water Fluoridation Act of 1985 to *require* water companies to fluoridate water supplies if requested to do so by the Health Authorities after they have undertaken all necessary consultative procedures.
- Give appropriate priority to, and make available adequate resources for, oral health promotion.
- Collect more data on groups known to be at a higher risk of dental caries, oral cancer and other oral diseases.
- In the absence of water fluoridation, consider other public health vehicles for fluoride.
- Include oral health benefits as part of the public education campaign on the dangers of smoking and excessive alcohol consumption.
- Consider strengthening present legislation restricting the advertising, sale and consumption of tobacco, and clarify legislation controlling the sale of cured chewing tobacco.

5 Recommendations to industry

5.1 *Water companies*

- Fluoridate water supplies when asked to do so by Health Authorities.

5.2 *Food manufacturers and retailers*

- Continue to increase choice and availability of affordable non-cariogenic snack foods/drinks.
- Adopt full nutrition labelling. In addition to information on energy, protein, carbohydrate and fat, information on sugars, saturates, fibre and sodium should be provided.

5.3 *Pharmaceutical companies*

- Continue to develop and make available sugar-free medicines.

5.4 *Oral healthcare product companies*

- Continue to improve the effectiveness of oral healthcare products.

6 Recommendations to healthcare (including dental) professionals

- Increase efforts to educate patients with consistent and effective advice and information on ways to improve oral health, in line with all the *Recommendations to individuals* above.
- Take opportunities for appropriate in-service training on oral health promotion.

7 Recommendations to dental professionals

- Utilise effective preventive technologies and oral health counselling for patients at risk of oral diseases.

8 Recommendations to schools/teachers

- Educate children about the importance of toothbrushing in relation to oral health.
- Educate children about the importance of diet in relation to oral health as well as general health.
- Provide and encourage the use of non-cariogenic snacks and drinks between meals.

GLOSSARY AND ABBREVIATIONS

Abrasion Wear of the tooth due to external physical forces such as toothbrushing.

Abscess Tissue cavity filled with pus; a response to local infection or damage.

Acidogenicity (1) Capacity of a food or drink, due to fermentation of its carbohydrate by bacteria, to result in the production of acid at the tooth surface; (2) the ability of bacteria to produce acid.

Acini Hollow clumps containing saliva-producing cells.

Adenoma A benign tumour of glandular epithelium.

Aerobe A microorganism requiring oxygen for growth.

Alveolar bone The bone which supports the teeth.

Ameloblasts Enamel-forming cells.

Amylase An enzyme present in saliva that breaks down starch molecules in food to sugars.

Anaemia Low haemoglobin concentration in the blood, sometimes due to inadequate supply of iron (iron deficiency anaemia).

Anaerobe A microorganism not requiring oxygen for growth (often killed by exposure to air [oxygen]).

Angular stomatitis see Angular cheilitis.

Angular cheilitis Inflammation of the lips at the corners of the mouth.

Aphthae Recurrent mouth ulcers.

Approximal surface Surface of a tooth which is adjacent to the next tooth in the same jaw.

Atrophy Thinning or wasting of a tissue.

Attrition Tooth wear due to contact between occlusal or approximal surfaces (during chewing or grinding).

Bruxism Grinding of the teeth.

BSPD British Society of Paediatric Dentistry.

Bulimia An eating disorder in which self-induced vomiting is practised; this can lead to erosion of teeth.

Bulla Blister.

Burning mouth syndrome A condition characterised by a scalded sensation inside the mouth.

Calculus Mineralised plaque (tartar).

Carcinoma Cancer. Malignant tumour.

Caries see Dental caries.

Cariogenic Having the ability to cause dental caries.

Cariostatic Factors that counter or contain the progression of dental caries.

Cementoblasts Cells that form cementum.

Cementum Layer of bone-like material covering the roots of the teeth.

CFU Colony forming units (of bacteria).

Commensal Harmless microorganism, part of the usual flora.

Crown Exposed section of tooth; the part above the gum margin.

DDE Developmental defects of enamel.

Deciduous dentition Primary (milk; first; baby) teeth.

Demineralisation Loss of minerals from the surface or subsurface of a tooth.

Dental caries (tooth decay) The gradual destruction of the tooth beginning at the surface, by the action of plaque bacteria producing acid from fermentable carbohydrate in food and drink.

Dental follicle A capsule in the jaw in which the developing tooth is situated.

Dental lamina A fold of epithelial band during early fetal life from which teeth develop.

Dental plaque A sticky film of bacteria attached to the tooth surface. May contain polysaccharide produced from the diet by the bacteria.

Dentate Having teeth.

Dentine Inner layer of the tooth. Hard material composing the bulk of the tooth, covered by enamel on the crown, and by the cementum of the root.

Demarcated opacity A white area on the surface of enamel with a clearly defined boundary from adjacent enamel.

Determinant Any factor such as an event or characteristic which brings about change in a health condition.

Diffuse opacity A white area on the surface of enamel with a poorly defined boundary.

Disaccharide A unit of two monosaccharides,

e.g. sucrose is a compound of glucose and fructose molecules.

DMFS   Decayed, missing or filled tooth surfaces. An index of the degree of individual dental caries damage to permanent teeth (dmfs is used for the primary teeth).

DMFT   Decayed, missing or filled teeth. An index used to express total dental caries experience in the permanent teeth (dmft is used for primary teeth).

Dysphagia   Difficulty in swallowing.

Dysplasia   Abnormal alteration in size, shape and organisation of the cells within the tissues .

Edentate   Having no teeth.

EHP   Enamel hypoplasia.

Embryogenesis   Formation of the embryo following fertilisation.

Enamel   Outer layer of the crown of the tooth; hardest substance in the body.

Epithelium   Layer of tissue covering the internal and external surfaces of the body.

Erosion (hard tissue)   The dissolution and softening of the tooth surface by acids, usually from food/drink. Usually accompanied or accelerated by abrasion and attrition.

Erosion (soft tissue)   An area of partial loss of thickness of the epithelium.

Erythroplakia   A pre-malignant red patch.

Exophytic   Proliferating on the exterior or surface epithelium of an organ or other structure in which the growth originated.

Extrinsic sugars   Sugars which are not contained within the cellular structure of foods.

Fermentable carbohydrate   Carbohydrate that oral bacteria are able to break down, resulting in the production of acid.

Flora   Microorganisms found in/on body sites (e.g. in the mouth).

Fluorosis   A defect of enamel mineralisation due to inappropriately high intakes of fluoride.

Geographic tongue   Migrating red patches of thin epithelium on the surface of the tongue.

Gingiva   Gum.

Gingivitis   Inflammation of the gingiva (gum).

Glossitis   Inflammation of the tongue.

GPPR   Gram-positive pleomorphic rods (usually Actinomyces species).

Hard tissues   Bone and teeth.

Histiogenesis   Formation of different tissues in individual organs in the fetus.

Hypercementosis   Deposition of additional cementum at the root of the tooth—this lengthens the tooth (usually occurs in older people).

Hyperkeratosis   An increase in the keratinisation of the epithelium.

Hypocalcaemia   A concentration of calcium in plasma which is below normal.

Hypoplasia   Under-development, e.g. of enamel.

Hyposalivation   Very low levels of saliva production.

Hypoxia   Depletion of oxygen.

ICD   (International Classification of Disease)   World Health Organisation disease classification code numbers.

In vitro   Experimental observation isolated from the whole body, e.g. in isolated cell or tissue taken from the body (literally 'in glass').

In vivo   Experimental observation in a living body.

In situ   Experiment using isolated tissue replaced in human body.

Incisors   Teeth at the front of the mouth with sharp cutting edges.

Index   An agreed set of criteria, standards or values used to record a disease. A method of counting or quantifying disease.

Intrinsic sugars   Sugars within the cellular structure of food.

Keratinisation   Production of keratin (a waxy substance) by epithelial cells.

Kelly-Paterson syndrome   (also Plummer-Vinson)   Disorder characterised by iron deficiency anaemia and resulting in difficulty in swallowing due to the formation of an oesophageal web.

Lactose   A disaccharide comprising glucose and galactose molecules.

LEHP   Linear enamel hypoplasia.

Linear enamel hypoplasia   Under-development of enamel which has occurred over a specific short time, resulting in a line of defective enamel of the tooth.

Leukoplakia   A white patch on the soft tissues of the mouth; often a precursor to cancerous changes.

Lichen planus   A skin disorder, often seen in the mouth as whitening and inflammation of the soft tissues.

Light-for-gestational age baby   A baby whose birthweight is well below that expected for the length of gestation, e.g. below the third centile of weight for gestational age in a reference population.

Low birthweight   Weight at birth less than 2500 g irrespective of the length of gestation.

Macronutrients   Nutrients consumed in large amounts, providing energy in the diet (fat, carbohydrate, protein).

Maltose   A disaccharide comprising two molecules of glucose.

Mandible   Lower jaw.

Mastication   Chewing.

Maxilla   Upper jaw.

Micronutrients   Vitamins and minerals.

Milk teeth see Deciduous dentition.

Mixed dentition stage When both deciduous and permanent teeth are present in the mouth.

Molars Teeth at the back of the mouth with a flat grinding surface.

Monosaccharide A single sugar molecule, e.g. glucose.

Mutans streptococci A group of bacteria which have been implicated in the development of caries.

Neoplasm A tumour (benign or malignant).

NMES Non-milk extrinsic sugars; all sugars outside the cellular structure of foods other than lactose in milk and milk products.

NSP Non-starch polysccharide (dietary fibre).

Nursing-bottle caries Particular pattern of rampant caries on the smooth surface of the front teeth seen in infants.

Occlusal surface Surface of a back tooth which meets opposing tooth in the other jaw.

Odontoblasts Dentine-forming cells.

Oligosaccharides A chain of between three and twenty monosaccharides.

Oral dysaesthesia An unpleasant sensation affecting the oral tissues.

Organogenesis Formation of organs in the fetus during the first three months (first trimester) of pregnancy.

Orthokeratinisation Complete surface keratinisation.

Papillae Small raised cones (filaments) on the tongue.

Parotid gland Saliva-producing gland in the cheek.

Pellicle Thin protein layer forming on the enamel surface; derived from proteins in saliva.

PEM Protein energy malnutrition.

Periodontitis Chronic inflammation of the periodontal ligament.

Periodontium Supporting structures of the teeth—cementum, periodontal ligament, gingivae and alveolar bone.

Permanent dentition Secondary (adult) teeth.

Pharynx Part of the alimentary canal between the mouth and the oesophagus.

Plaque see Dental plaque.

Plummer-Vinson syndrome see Kelly-Paterson syndrome.

Polysaccharides Complex carbohydrates usually containing 20 or more monosaccharides.

ppm Part per million (also mg/l).

Predentine Dentine prior to mineralisation.

Preterm baby A baby born at less than 37 weeks of gestation, irrespective of birthweight.

Primary teeth Deciduous teeth.

Pulp The blood vessels and nerve tissue in the centre of the tooth.

Rampant caries Rapidly progressing decay involving tooth surfaces not usually affected.

Recurrent aphthae Recurrent ulcers in the mouth which heal spontaneously and are limited to the non-keratinising moveable soft tissues.

Remineralisation A return of minerals to the surface of the tooth after demineralisation.

Rete pegs Projections from the inner layer of the epithelium into the underlying tissue.

Root Section of tooth below the gum not covered by enamel. The roots of teeth may be exposed as a result of gum disease.

Secondary teeth See permanent dentition.

Sialadenitis Inflammation of the salivary glands.

Sialosis Benign enlargement of the salivary glands.

Sjögren's syndrome A condition characterised by dry eyes and dry mouth either alone (primary form), or with a connective tissue disorder (secondary form).

Soft palate Part at the back of the palate without underlying bone.

Soft tissues Gum, tongue, glands and lining of the lips and cheeks.

Sorbitol A sugar-alcohol used as a bulk sweetener in foods; a hydrogenated hexose sugar.

Stomatitis Inflammation of the mouth.

Sublingual gland Saliva-producing gland under the tongue.

Submandibular gland Saliva-producing gland in the floor of the mouth.

Sucrose A disaccharide comprising glucose and fructose.

Sugar alcohol Bulk sweetener derived from monosaccharides or disaccharides by reduction (hydrogenation) of an aldehyde or ketone group to an alcohol group.

Sugars Any mono- or disaccharide.

Sulcus The crevice between the tooth and the gum.

Tartar see Calculus.

TF index A index of fluorosis developed by Thylstrup and Fejerskov.

Tooth wear Loss of tooth substance; tooth-tissue loss; abrasion, attrition and/or erosion.

TSIF Total surface index of fluorosis.

Ulceration A breach in the epithelial surface.

White spot An early carious lesion on the tooth where enamel is demineralised but the surface is still intact.

Wisdom teeth Third molars; usually erupt between 18–25 years of age behind the other teeth.

Xerostomia Dryness of the mouth.

Xylitol A bulk sweetner used in the production of 'tooth friendly' confectionery; a hydrogenated pentose sugar.

REFERENCES

Abrahams R (1983) Ethnic and religious aspects of diet. In *Nutrition and Pregnancy* (eds J McFadyen, J MacVicar). Royal College of Obstetricians and Gynaecologists, London, 23–29.

Abrams RA, Ruff JC (1986) Oral signs and symptoms in the diagnosis of bulimia. *J Am Dent Assoc* **113**, 761–64.

Agerberg G, Carlsson GE (1981) Chewing ability in relation to general and dental health. *Acta Odontologica Scandinavica* **39**, 147–153.

Al-Alousi W, Jackson D, Crompton G, Jenkins OC (1975) Enamel mottling in a fluoridated and a non-fluoridated community. *Brit Dent J* **138**, 9–15.

Alvarez JO, Caceda J, Woolley TW *et al.* (1993) A longitudinal study of dental caries in the primary teeth of children who suffered from infant malnutrition. *J Dent Res* **72**, 1573–1576.

Alvarez JO, Navia JM (1989) Nutritional status, tooth eruption and dental caries: A review. *Am J Clin Nutr* **49**, 417–426.

Ambjornsen E (1986) Decayed, missing and filled teeth among elderly people in a Norwegian municipality. *Acta Odontologica Scandinavica* **44**, 123–130.

American Dental Association (1986) Proceedings: Conference of methods of assessment of the cariogenic potential of foods. *J Dent Res* **65**, 1473–1543.

Anaise JZ (1980) Prevalence of dental caries among workers in the sweets industry in Israel. *Comm Dent Oral Epidemiol* **8**, 142–145.

Anderson RJ (1969) The relationship between dental conditions and the trace element molybdenum. *Caries Res* **3**, 75–87.

Andreen I, Kohler B (1992) Effects of Weight Watchers' diet on salivary secretion rate, buffer effect and numbers of mutans streptococci and lactobacilli. *Scand J Dent Res* **100**, 93–97.

Angmar-Mansonn B, Whitford GM (1990) Environmental and physiological factors affecting dental fluorosis. *J Dent Res* **68**, S706–S713.

Anonymous (1985) World population prospects. Estimates and projections in 1982. In *United Nations DIFSA Populations Studies*, Vol. 86. United Nations, New York.

Aponte-Merced L, Navia JM (1980) Pre-eruptive protein malnutrition and acid solubility of rat molar enamel surfaces. *Arch Oral Biol* **25**, 701–705.

Assev S, Scheie AA (1986) Xylitol metabolism in xylitol sensitive and xylitol resistant strains of streptococci. *Acta Pathol Microbiol Immunol Scand* B. **94**, 239–243.

Atwal GS (1995) Betel-quid (pan) chewing amongst Asians living in London. MSc Thesis, University of London.

Aukett A, Wharton B (1989) Nutrition of Asian children: infants and toddlers. In *Ethnic Factors in Health and Disease* (eds JK Cruickshank, DG Beevers). Wright, London.

Averill HM, Averill JE (1968) The effect of daily apple consumption on dental caries experience, oral hygiene status and upper respiratory infections. *NY State Dent J* **34**, 403–409.

Axéll T (1987) Occurrence of leukoplakia and some other oral white lesions among 20,333 adult Swedish people. *Comm Dent Oral Epidemiol* **15**, 46–51.

Baird IM, Dodge OG, Palmer FJ, Wawman RJ (1961) The tongue and oesophagus in iron deficiency anaemia and the effect of iron therapy. *J Clin Pathol* **14**, 603–609.

Baker KA, Didcock EA, Kemm JR, Patrick JM (1983) Effect of age, sex and illness on salt taste detection thresholds. *Age & Ageing* **12**, 159–165.

Balarajan R, Raleigh VS (1992) The ethnic populations of England and Wales: the 1991 census. *Health Trends* **24**, 113–116.

Bánóczy J (1977) Follow-up studies in oral leukoplakia. *J Maxillofacial Surg* **5**, 69–75.

Bánóczy J, Rigo O (1991) Prevalence study of oral precancerous lesions within a complex screening system in Hungary. *Comm Dent Oral Epidemiol* **19**, 265–267.

Barclay A (1851) Death from anaemia. *Medical Times Gazette* **23**, 480–482.

Barra S, Franceschi S, Negri E *et al.* (1990) Type of alcoholic beverage and cancer of the oral cavity, pharynx and oesophagus in an Italian area with high wine consumption. *Int J Canc* **46**,1017–1020.

Baum BJ (1986) Salivary gland function during ageing. *Gerodontics* **2**, 61–64.

Beckers HJ, van der Hoeven JS (1984) The effects of mutual interaction and host diet on the growth rates of the bacteria *Actinomyces viscosus* and *Streptococcus mutans* during colonization of tooth surfaces in di-associated gnotobiotic rats. *Arch Oral Biol* **29**, 231–236.

Bedi R, Elton R (1991) The dental health of Asian schoolchildren attending Glasgow and Trafford schools. *Commun Dental Health* **8**, 17–23.

Bedi R, Gilthorpe MS (1995) Betel-quid and tobacco chewing among the Bangladeshi community in areas of multiple deprivation. In *Betel-quid and Tobacco Chewing among the Bangladeshi Community in the United Kingdom. Usage and Health Issues* (eds R Bedi, P Jones). Centre for Transcultural Oral Health, London, 37–52.

Bedi R, Quarrell I, Kippen A (1991) The dental health of ten year children attending multiracial schools in Greater Glasgow. *Brit Dent J* **170**, 182–185.

Bedi R, Uppal RDK (1995) The oral health of minority ethnic communities in the United Kingdom. *Brit Dent J* **179**, 421–425.

Beighton D (1993) A microbiological study of primary root caries lesions with different treatment needs. *J Dent Res* **72**, 623–629.

Beighton D, Adamson A, Rugg-Gunn A (1996) Associations between dietary intake, dental caries experience and salivary bacterial levels in 12-year-old English schoolchildren. *Arch Oral Biol* **41**, 271–280.

Beighton D, Carr AD, Oppenheim BA (1994) Identification of viridans streptococci associated with bacteraemia in neutropenic cancer patients. *J Med Microbiol* **40**, 202–204.

Beighton D, Hardie JM, Whiley RA (1991a) A scheme for the identification of viridans streptococci. *J Med Microbiol* **35**, 367–372.

Beighton D, Hayday H, Walker J (1985) The relationship between the number of bacterium *Streptococcus mutans* at discreet sites on the dentition of macaque monkeys (*Macaca fascicularis*) and the subsequent development of dental caries. *Arch Oral Biol* **30**, 85–88.

Beighton D, Hayday H (1986) The influence of diet on the growth of streptococcal bacteria on the molar teeth of monkeys (*Macaca fascicularis*). *Arch Oral Biol* **31**, 449–454.

Beighton D, Hellyer PH, Lynch EJ, Heath MR (1991b) Salivary levels of mutans streptococci, lactobacilli, yeasts, and root caries prevalence in non-institutionalised elderly dental patients. *Comm Dent Oral Epidemiol* **19**, 302–307.

Beighton D, Ludford R, Clark DT et al. (1995) Use of CHROMagar Candida medium for the isolation of yeasts from dental samples. *J Clin Microbiol* **33**, 3025–3027.

Beighton D, Lynch E (1995) Comparison of selected microflora of plaque and underlying carious dentine associated with primary root caries lesions. *Caries Res* **29**, 154–158.

Beighton D, Russell RR, Whiley RA (1991) A simple biochemical scheme for the differentiation of *Streptococcus mutans* and *Streptococcus sobrinus*. *Caries Res* **25**, 174–178.

Beighton D, Smith K, Hayday H (1986) The growth of bacteria and the production of exoglycosidic enzymes in the dental plaque of macaque monkeys. *Arch Oral Biol* **31**, 829–835.

Bender DA (1993) *Introduction to Nutrition and Metabolism*. University College London Press, London.

Bennett N, Dodd T, Flatley J, Freeth S, Balling K (1995) *Health Survey for England 1993*. HMSO, London.

Bentovim D, Morton J (1990) The epidemiology of anorexia nervosa in South Australia. *Australian & New Zealand J Psychiat* **24**, 182–198.

Bergman KE, Bergman RL (1995) Salt fluoridation and general health. *Adv Dent Res* **9**, 138–143.

Berkowitz RJ, Jordan HV, White G (1975) The early establishment of *Streptococcus mutans* in the mouths of infants. *Arch Oral Biol* **20**, 171–174.

Beveridge BR, Bannerman RM, Evanson JM, Witts LJ (1965b) Hypochromic anaemia. A retrospective study and follow-up of 378 patients. *Quart J Med* **34**, 145–161.

Bibby BG (1983) Fruits and vegatables and dental caries. *Clin Prevent Dent* **5**, 3–11.

Birkhed D, Bar A (1991) Sorbitol and dental caries. *World Rev Nutr and Diet* **65**, 1–37.

Blinkhorn AS (1982) The caries experience and dietary habits of Edinburgh nursery school children. *Brit Dent J* **152**, 227–230.

Blot WJ, McLaughlin JK, Winn DM (1988) Smoking and drinking in relation to oral and pharyngeal cancer. *Cancer Res* **48**, 3282–3287.

Bochud PY, Calandra T, Francioli P (1994) Bacteremia due to viridans streptococci in neutropenic patients: a review. *Am J Med* **97**, 256–264.

Boffetta P, Mashberg A, Winkelman R, Garfinkel L (1992) Carcinogenic effect of tobacco smoking and alcohol drinking on anatomic sites of the oral cavity and oropharynx. *Int J Canc* **52**, 530–533.

Booth IW (1992) Silent gastro-oesophageal reflux: how much do we miss. *Arch Disease Childh* **67**, 1325–1327.

Bouquot JE, Gorlin RJ (1986) Leukoplakia, lichen planus, and other oral keratoses in 23,616 white Americans over the age of 35 years. *Oral Surg* **61**, 373–381.

Bouvet AA, Durand C, Devine J, Etienne C, Leport (Group d'Enquêtte sur l'Endocarditie en France en 1990, 1991, 1994) In vitro suspectibility to antibiotics of 200 strains of streptococci and enterococci isolated during infective endocarditis. In *Pathogenic Streptococci: Present and Future* (ed A. Totolian). Lancer Publications, St. Petersburg, Russia, 72–73.

Bovina C, Landi L, Pasquali P, Marchetti M (1969) Biosynthesis of folate coenzymes in riboflavin deficient rats. *J Nutr* **99**, 320–324.

Bowden GH (1990) Microbiology of root surface lesions in humans. *J Dent Res* **69**, 1205–1210.

Bowden GH, Ekstrand J, McNaughton B, Challacombe SJ (1990) Association of selected bacteria with the lesions of root surface caries. *Oral Microbiol Immunol* **5**, 346–351.

Bowen WH (1981) Dental caries in primates. In *Animal Models in Cariology* (ed JM Tanzer). IRL, London, 131–135.

Bowen WH, Amsbaugh SM, Monell-Torrens S et al. (1980) A method to assess cariogenic potential of foodstuffs. *J Am Dent Assoc* **100**, 677–681.

Boyar RM, Thylstrup A, Holmen L, Bowden GH (1989) The microflora associated with the development of initial enamel decalcification below orthodontic bands in vivo in children living in a fluoridated water area. *J Dent Res* **68**, 1734–1738.

Braddon FEM, Wadsworth MEJ, Davies JMC, Cripps HA (1988) Social and regional differences in food and alcohol consumption and their measurement in a national birth cohort. *J Epidemiol Commun Health* **42**, 341–349.

Bradnock G, Marchment MD, Anderson RJ (1984) Social background, fluoridation and caries experience in a 5-year-old population in the West Midlands. *Brit Dent J* **156**, 127–131.

Bradshaw DJ, Homer KA, Marsh PD, Beighton D (1994) Metabolic cooperation in oral microbial communities during growth on mucin. *Microbiology* **140**, 3407–3412.

Bramstedt F (1975) Teeth and nutrition. *Bibliotheca Nutritio et Dieta* 1–16.

Bratthall D, Hansel-Petersson G, Sundberg H (1996) Reasons for the caries decline: what do the experts believe? *Eur J Oral Sci* **104**, 416–422.

Brice DM, Blum JR, Steinberg BJ (1996) The aetiology, treatment and prevention of nursing caries. *Compend Cont Ed Dent* **17**, 92, 94, 96–98.

Bridgman C (1993) Morbidity following general anaesthesia for exodontia. MSc Thesis, University of Liverpool.

British Dental Association (BDA), British Society of Paediatric Dentistry and British Association for the Study of Community Dentistry (1997) Fluoride supplement dosage. *Brit Dent J* **182**, 6–7.

British Fluoridation Society (BFS) (1995). *One in a Million*. University of Liverpool, School of Dentistry, Liverpool.

BFS (1997) *Dental Health Inequalities in the United Kingdom*. British Fluoridation Society Briefing Paper.

British Nutrition Foundation (BNF) (1995) *Iron: Nutritional and Physiological Significance*. Chapman & Hall, London.

British Society of Paediatric Dentistry (BSPD) (1995) A policy document on toothfriendly sweets. *Int J Paediat Dent* **5**, 195–197.

BSPD (1996) A policy document on fluoride dietary supplements and fluoride toothpaste for children. *Int J Paediat Dent* **6**, 139–142.

British Soft Drinks Association (1991, 1995) *Consumption Figures*. British Soft Drinks Association, 22 Stukeley Street, London, WC2B 5LR.

Brook AH, Fearne JM, Smith JM (1997) Environmental causes of enamel defects. In *Dental Enamel*. John Wiley, Chichester, 212–240.

Brown C (1984) *Black and White Britain: The Third PSI Survey*. Heinemann, London.

Brown JP (1980) The efficacy and economy of comprehensive dental care for handicapped children. *Int Dent J* **30**, 14–27.

Brugere J, Quenel P, Leclerc A, Rodriguez J (1986) Differential effects of tobacco and alcohol in cancer of the larynx, pharynx and mouth. *Cancer* **57**, 391–395.

Budtz Jorgensen E, Stenderup A, Grabowski M (1975) An epidemiological study of yeasts in elderly denture wearers. *Comm Dent Oral Epidemiol* **3**, 115–119.

Burt BA, Ismail AI (1986) Diet, nutrition, and food cariogenicity. *J Dent Res* **65**, S1475–S1484.

Burt BA, Eklund SA, Morgan KL *et al.* (1988) The effects of sugars intake and frequency of ingestion on dental caries increment in a three-year longitudinal study. *J Dent Res* **67**, 1422–1429.

Cancer Research Campaign (1993) *Oral Cancer*, Factsheet 14. CRC, London.

Carlos JP (1987) *Oral Health of United States Adults*. National Institute of Dental Research Survey of Adult Oral Health, National Institutes of Health, Maryland.

Carlos JP, Wolfe MD (1989). Methodological and nutritional issues in assessing the oral health of aged subjects. *Am J Clin Nutr* **50**, 1210–1218; discussion 1231–1235.

Carlsson GE (1984) The effect of age, the loss of teeth and prosthetic rehabilitation. *Int Dent J* **34**, 93–97.

Carlsson J, Herrmann BF, Hofling JF, Sundqvist GK (1984) Degradation of the human proteinase inhibitors alpha-1-antitrypsin and alpha-2-macroglobulin by *Bacteroides gingivalis*. *Infect Immun* **43**, 644–648.

Carmichael CL, French AD, Rugg-Gunn AJ, Furness JA (1980) The effect of fluoridation upon the relationship between caries experience and social class in 5-year-old children in Newcastle and Northumberland. *Brit Dent J* **149**, 163–167.

Carmichael CL, Rugg-Gunn AJ, Ferrell RS (1989) The relationship between fluoridation, social class and caries experience in 5-year-old children in Newcastle and Northumberland. *Brit Dent J* **167**, 57–61.

Central Statistical Office (1996). *A Report of the 1995–1996 Family Expenditure Survey*. HMSO, London.

Cerklewski FL (1981) Effect of suboptimal zinc nutrition during gestation and lactation on rat molar tooth composition and dental caries. *J Nutr* 1780–1783.

Cerna H, Fiala B, Fingerova H, Pohanka E, Szwarcon A (1984). Contribution to indication of total therapy with vitamin E in chronic periodontal disease (pilot study). *Acta Universitatis Palackianae Olomucensis Facultatis Medicae* **107**, 167–170.

Chapman G, Maclean H (1993) 'Junk food' and 'healthy food': meanings of food in adolescent women's culture. *J Nutr Ed* **25**, 108–113.

Chauhan J, Hawrysh ZJ, Gee M, Donald EA, Basu TK (1987) Age-related olfactory and taste changes and interrelationships between taste and nutrition. *J Am Diet Assoc* **87**, 1543–1550.

Chief Justice O'Dalaigh (1964). Fluoridation. Judgement of the Supreme Court of Ireland delivered by Chief Justice O'Dalaigh, 3 July, 1964. Department of Health: Dublin.

Chisholm M, Ardran GM, Callender ST, Wright R (1971) Iron deficiency and autoimmunity in postcricoid webs. *Quart J Med* **40**, 421–433.

Clancy KL, Bibby BG, Goldberg HJV *et al.* (1977) *Snack food intake of adolescents and caries development*. *J Dent Res* **45**, 568–573.

Clark DW (1985) Oral complications of anorexia nervosa and/or bulimia. *J Oral Med* **40**, 134–138.

Clarkson J (1989) Review of terminology, classification and indices of developmental defects of enamel. *Adv Dent Res* **3**, 104–109.

Clarkson BH (1986) *In vitro* methods for testing the cariogenic potential of foods. *J Dent Res* **65**, 1516–1519.

Cockburn F, Belton NR, Purvis RJ *et al*. (1980) Maternal vitamin D intake and mineral metabolism in mothers and their newborn infants. *Brit Med J* **ii**, 11–14.

Coleman D, Salt J (1996) The ethnic group question in the 1991 census: a new landmark in British social statistics. In *Ethnicity in the 1991 Census*, Vol. 1. (eds D Coleman, J. Salt). HMSO, London.

Cooke WT, Holmes GKT (1984) *Coeliac Disease*. Churchill Livingstone, Edinburgh.

Corbett ME, Moore WJ (1976) Distribution of dental caries in ancient British populations IV: the 19th century. *Caries Res* **10**, 401–414.

Coumoulos H, Mellanby M (1947) Dental condition of five-year old children in institutions and private schools compared with LCC schools. *Brit Med J* **i**, 751–756.

Curzon MEJ (1983) Strontium. In *Trace Elements and Dental Disease* (eds MEJ Curzon, TE Cutress). John Wright, Boston.

Curzon MEJ, Cuttress TE (eds) (1983) *Trace Elements and Dental Disease*. John Wright, Boston.

Curzon MEJ, Pollard MA (1997) Do we still care about children's teeth? *Brit Dent J* **182**, 242–244.

Davies RM, Holloway PJ, Ellwood RP (1995) The role of fluoride dentifrices in a national strategy for the oral health of children. *Brit Dent J* **179**, 84–87.

de Soet JJ, van Loveren C, Lammens AJ *et al*. (1991) Differences in cariogenicity between fresh isolates of *Streptococcus sobrinus* and *Streptococcus mutans*. *Caries Res* **25**, 116–122.

de Soet JJ, Weerheijm KL, van Amerongen WE, de Graaff J (1995) A comparison of the microbiol flora in carious dentine of clinically detectable and undetectable occlusal lesions. *Caries Res* **29**, 46–49.

De Vries N, van Zandwijk N, Patorino U (1992) Chemoprevention in the management of oral cancer: Euroscan and other studies. *Eur J Canc* **28B**, 153–157.

Dent CE, Gupta MM (1975) Plasma 25-hydroxyvitamin D levels during pregnancy in Caucasians and in vegetarian and non vegetarian Asians. *Lancet* **ii**, 1057–1060.

Department of Health and Social Security (1985) *Fluoridation of Water and Cancer: A Review of the Epidemiological Evidence*. HMSO, London.

Department of Health (DH) (1989) Committee on Medical Aspects of Food Policy. *Dietary Sugars and Human Disease*. Report on Health and Social Subjects, No 37. HMSO, London.

DH (1991) Committee on Medical Aspects of Food Policy. *Dietary Reference Values for Food Energy and Nutrients for the United Kingdom*. Report on Health and Social Subjects, No 41. HMSO, London.

DH (1994) Committee on Medical Aspects of Food Policy. *Weaning and the Weaning Diet*. Report on Health and Social Subjects, No 45. HMSO, London.

Dicks LM, Du Plessis EM, Dellaglio F, Lauer E (1996) Reclassification of *Lactobacillus casei* subsp. *casei* ATCC 393 and *Lactobacillus rhamnosus* ATCC 15820 as *Lactobacillus zeae* nom. rev., designation of ATCC 334 as the neotype of *L. casei* subsp. *casei*, and rejection of the name *Lactobacillus paracasei*. *Int J Syst Bacteriol* **46**, 337–340.

Diorio LP, Miller SA, Navia JM (1973) The separate effects of protein and calorie malnutrition in the development and growth of rat bones and teeth. *J Nutr* **103**, 856–865.

Dobson B, Beardsworth A, Keil T, Walker R (1994) *Diet, Choice and Poverty*. Family Policy Studies Centre, London.

Doll R (1992) The lessons of life: keynote address to the nutrition and cancer conference. *Cancer Res* **52**, 2024–2029.

Douglas CW, Heath J, Hampton KK, Preston FE (1993) Identity of viridans streptococci isolated from cases of infective endocarditis. *J Med Microbiol* **39**, 179–182.

Dowell TB, Joyston-Bechal S (1981) Fluoride supplements—age related dosages. *Brit Dent J* **150**, 273–275.

Dowler E, Calvert C (1995) *Nutrition and Diet in Lone-Parent Families in London*. Family Policy Studies Centre, London..

Downer MC (1992) Time trends in caries experience in children in England and Wales. *Caries Res* **26**, 466–472.

Downer MC (1994) Caries prevalence in the United Kingdom. *Int Dent J* **44**, 365–370.

Downer MC (1996) The caries decline—a comment in light of the UK experience. *Eur J Oral Sci* **104**, 433–435.

Downer MC, Blinkhorn AS, Holt RD *et al*. (1994) Dental caries experience and defects of dental enamel among 12-year-old children in north London, Edinburgh, Glasgow and Dublin. *Comm Dent Oral Epidemiol* **22**, 283–285.

Dreizen S, Levy BM (1969) Histopathology of experimentally induced nutritional deficiency cheilosis in the marmoset (Callithrix jacchus). *Arch Oral Biol* **14**, 577–582.

Duchin S, van Houte J (1978) Relationship of *Streptococcus mutans* and lactobacilli to incipient smooth surface caries in man. *Arch Oral Biol* **23**, 779–786.

Duggal MS, Curzon MEJ (1989) An evaluation of the cariogenic potential of baby and infant fruit drinks. *Brit Dent J* **166**, 327–330.

Duxbury JT, Lennon MA, Mitropoulos CM, Worthington HV (1987) Differences in caries levels in 5-year-old children in Newcastle and North Manchester in 1985. *Brit Dent J* **162**, 457–458.

Edgar WM, Bibby BG, Mundorff S, Rowley J (1975) Acid production in plaques after eating snacks: modifying factors in foods. *J Am Dent Assoc* **90**, 418–425.

Einhorn J, Wersäll J (1967) Incidence of oral carcinoma in patients with leukoplakia of the oral cavity. *Cancer* **20**, 2189–2193.

Eisenberg AD (1983) Lithium. In *Trace Elements and Dental Disease* (eds MEJ Curzon, TE Cutress). John Wright, Boston.

Ekstrand J, Spak CJ, Vogel G (1990) Pharmacokinetics of fluoride in man and its clinical relevance. *J Dent Res* **69**, S550–S555.

Ellen RP, Banting DW, Fillery ED (1985) Longitudinal microbiological investigation of a hospitalised population of older adults with a high root surface caries risk. *J Dent Res* **64**, 1377–1381.

Ellwood RP, O'Mullane DM (1995) Dental enamel opacities in three groups with varying levels of fluoride in their drinking water. *Caries Res* **29**, 137–142.

Elwood JM, Pearson JCG, Skippen DH, Jackson SM (1984) Alcohol, smoking, social and occupational factors in the aetiology of cancer of the oral cavity, pharynx and larynx. *Int J Canc* **34**, 603–612.

Enwonwu CO (1973) Influence of socio-economic conditions on dental development in Nigerian children. *Arch Oral Biol* **18**, 95–107.

Ericsson Y, Forsman B (1969) Fluoride retained from mouthrinses and dentifrices in pre-school children. *Caries Res* **3**, 290–299.

Evans DJ (1991) A study of developmental defects in enamel in 10-year-old high social class children residing in a non-fluoridated area. *Commun Dent Health* **8**, 31–38.

Evans DJ, Rugg-Gunn AJ, Tabari ED, Butler T (1996) The effect of fluoridation and social class on caries experience in 5-year-old Newcastle children in 1994 compared with results over the previous 18 years. *Commun Dent Health* **13**, 5–10.

FAO/WHO (1997) *Carbohydrates in Human Nutrition. Interim Report of a Joint FAO/WHO Expert Consultation (14 to 18 April 1997)*. Food and Agricultural Organisation, Rome.

Farrell JH (1956) The effect of mastication on the digestion of food. *Brit Dent J* **100**, 149–155.

Farrell JH (1957) Partial dentures in the restoration of masticatory efficiency. *Dent Pract Dent Rec* **7**, 375–379.

Fearne JM, Bryan EM, Elliman AM, Brook AH, Williams DM (1990) Enamel defects in the primary dentition of children born weighing less than 2000 g. *Brit Dent J* **168**, 433–437.

Federation Dentaire Internationale (FDI) (1982) An epidemiological index of developmental defects of dental enamel (DDE Index) *Int Dent J* **32**, 251–259.

FDI (1992) A review of the developmental defects of enamel index (DDE Index). Commission on Oral Heath, Research & Epidemiology. *Int Dent J* **42**, 11–426.

Fejerskov O, Manji F, Baelum V, Moller IJ (1988) *Dental Fluorosis—A Handbook for Health Workers*. Munksgaard, Copenhagen.

Ferguson MM (1975) Oral mucous membrane markers of internal disease: disorders of the endocrine system, haemopoietic system and nutrition. In *Oral Mucosa in Health and Disease* (ed AE Dolby). Oxford, 233–299.

Ferguson MM, Dagg JH (1974) Oral ulceration due to ascorbic acid deficiency. *Lancet* **1**, 164.

Fernald GW, Roberts MW, Boat TF (1990) Cystic fibrosis: a current review. *Pediat Dent* **12**, 72–78.

Firestone AR, Schmid R, Muhlemann HR (1982) Cariogenic effects of cooked wheat starch alone or with sucrose and frequency-controlled feedings in rats. *Arch Oral Biol* **27**, 759–763.

Fisher FJ (1968) A field survey of dental caries,

periodontal disease and enamel defects in Tristan da Cunha. *Brit Dent J* **125**, 447–453.

Foy H, Kondi A, Mbaya V (1966) Serum vitamin B12 and folate levels in normal and riboflavin deficient baboons. *Brit J Haematol* **12**, 239–245.

Franceschi S, Talamini R, Barra S et al. (1990). Smoking and drinking in relation to cancers of the oral cavity, pharynx, larynx and esophagus in Northern Italy. *Cancer Res* **50**, 6502–6507.

Franco EL, Kowalski LP, Oliveira BV et al. (1989) Risk factors for oral cancer in Brazil: a case-control study. *Int J Canc* **43**, 992–1000.

Frandsen EV, Pedrazzoli V, Kilian M (1991) Ecology of viridans streptococci in the oral cavity and pharynx. *Oral Microbiol Immunol* **6**, 129–133.

Frick HF, Kummer B, Putz RV (ed.) (1990) *Wolf–Heidegger's Atlas of Human Anatomy*, 4th edn. Karger AG, Basel.

Galagan DJ (1953) Climate and controlled fluoridation. *J Am Dent Assoc* **47**, 159–170.

Galan D, Lynch E (1993) Epidemiology of root caries. *Gerodontology* **10**, 59–71.

Gandara BK, Izutsu KT, Truelove EL (1985) Age-related salivary flow rate changes in controls and patients with oral lichen planus. *J Dent Res* **64**, 1149–1151.

Gedalia I, Dakuar A, Shapira L, Leminstein I, Goultschin J, Rahamin E (1991a) Enamel softening with coca-cola and rehardening with milk or saliva. *Am J Dent* **4**, 120–122.

Gedalia I, Lonat-Bendat D, Ben-Moshek S, Shapira L (1991b) Tooth enamel softening with a cola type drink and rehardening with hard cheese or stimulated saliva *in situ*. *J Oral Rehab* **18**, 501–506.

Gibbons RJ (1996) Role of adhesion in microbial colonization of host tissues: a contribution of oral microbiology. *J Dent Res* **75**, 866–870.

Gibson J, Stassen LFA, Lamey P, Fell GS (1990) Geographic tongue: the clinical response to zinc supplementation. *J Trace Elements in Exper Med* **3**, 203–208.

Gillman, T (1970) *An Introduction to the Biology of the Skin* (eds RH Champion, T Gillman, AJ Rook, RT Sims). Blackwell Science, Oxford.

Gislen G, Nilsson KO, Matsson L (1980) Gingival inflammation in diabetic children related to degree of metabolic control. *Acta Odontologica Scandinavica* **38**, 241–246.

Glickman I (1979) Nutritional influences on the periodontum. In *Glickman's Clinical Periodontology*, 5th edn. Saunders, Philadelphia, 489–505.

Godson JH, Williams SA, Kwan S (1996) Inter-generational changes in diet, growth and oral health among a 3-year-old Muslim population in England. *Scand J Nutr* **40**, 114–118.

Godson JH, Williams SA (1996) Oral health and health related behaviours among three-year-old children born to first and second generation Pakistani mothers in Bradford, UK. *Commun Dent Health* **13**, 27–33.

Goodson J M, Bowles D (1973) The effect of α-tocopherol on sulcus fluid flow in periodontal disease. *J Dent Res* **52**, 217.

Graham S, Dayal H, Rohrer T et al. (1977) Dentition,

diet, tobacco and alcohol in the epidemiology of oral cancer. *J Nat Can Inst* **59**, 1611–1618.

Grahnen H, Holm AK, Magnusson B, Sjölin S. (1972) Mineralization defects of the primary teeth in intrauterine undernutrition. *Caries Res* **6**, 224–228.

Gratrix D, Holloway PJ (1994) Factors of deprivation associated with dental caries in young children. *Commun Dent Health* **11**, 66–70.

Grbic JT, Lamster IB (1991) Risk indicators for future periodontal attachment loss in adult periodontitis. Patient variables. *J Periodontol* **62**, 322–329.

Grbic JT, Lamster IB (1992) Risk indicators for future periodontal attachement loss in adult periodontitis. Tooth and site variables. *J Periodontol* **63**, 262–269.

Gregory JR, Collins DL, Davies PSW et al. (1995) *National Diet and Nutrition Survey: Children Aged $1\frac{1}{2}$ to $4\frac{1}{2}$ Years*, Vol. 1: *Report of the Diet and Nutrition Survey*. HMSO, London.

Gregory J, Foster K, Tyler H, Wiseman M (1990) *The Dietary and Nutritional Survey of British Adults*. HMSO, London.

Grenby T (1990) Snack foods and dental caries. Investigations using laboratory animals. *Brit Dent J* **168**, 353–360.

Grindefjord M, Dahllof G, Modeer T (1995a) Caries development in children from 2.5 to 3.5 years of age: a longitudinal study. *Caries Res* **29**, 449–454.

Grindefjord M, Dahllof G, Nilsson B, Modeer T (1995b) Prediction of dental caries development in 1 year old children. *Caries Res* **29**, 343–348.

Grindefjord M, Dahllof G, Nilsson B, Modeer T (1996) Stepwise prediction of dental caries in children up to 3.5 years of age. *Caries Res* **30**, 256–266.

Grobler SR, Blignaut JB (1989) The effect of a high consumption of apples or grapes on dental caries and periodontal disease in humans. *Clin Prevent Dent* **11**, 8–12.

Groeneveld A, van Eck AAMJ, Backer Dirks O (1990) Fluoride in caries prevention: is the effect pre- or post-eruptive? *J Dent Res* **69**, S751-S755.

Grytten J, Rossow I, Holst D, Steele L (1988) Longitudinal study of dental health behaviours and other caries predictors in early childhood. *Comm Dent Oral Epidemiol* **16**, 356–359.

Grzegorczyk PB, Jones SW, Mistretta CM (1979) Age-related differences in salt taste acuity. *J Gerontol* **34**, 834–840.

Guha-Chowdhury N, Drummond BW, Smillie AC (1996) Total fluoride intake in children aged 3–4 years—a longitudinal study. *J Dent Res* **75**, 1451–1457.

Gunne HJ (1985a) The effect of removable partial dentures on mastication and dietary intake. *Acta Odontologica Scandinavica* **43**, 262–278.

Gunne HJ (1985b) Masticatory efficency and dental state. *Acta Odontologica Scandinavica* **43**, 139–146.

Günther S (1972a) Vitamin A acid in treatment of oral lichen planus. *Arch Dermatol* **106**, 854–857.

Günther S (1972b) Topical administration of vitamin A acid in palmar keratoses; callosities, hyperkeratotic eczema, hypertrophic lichen planus, pityriasis rubra pilaris. *Dermatologica* **145**, 344–347.

Gustafsson BE, Quensel CE, Lanke LS et al. (1954) The Vipeholm dental caries study. The effect of different levels of carbohydrate intake on caries activity in 436 individuals observed for five years. *Acta Odontologica Scandinavica* **11**, 232–364.

Hardie JM, Thomson PL, South RJ et al. (1977) A longitudinal epidemiological study on dental plaque and the development of dental caries—interim results after two years. *J Dent Res* **56**, C90-C98.

Hargreaves JA, Thompson GW (1989) Ultra-violet light and dental caries in children. *Caries Res* **23**, 389–392.

Harper DS, Abelson DC, Jensen ME (1986) Human plaque acidity models. *J Dent Res* **65**, 1503–1510.

Harris SS, Navia JM (1980) Vitamin A deficiency and caries susceptibility of rat molars. *Arch Oral Biol* **25**, 415–421.

Harris R (1963) Biology of the children of Hopewell House, Bowral, Australia. Observations on dental caries experience extending over 5 years (1957–61). *J Dent Res* **42**, 1387–1399.

Haugejorden O (1996) Using the DMF gender difference to assess the 'major' role of fluoride toothpastes in the caries decline in industrialized countries: a meta-analysis. *Comm Dent Oral Epidemiol* **24**, 369–375.

Hawley GM, Hamilton FA, Worthington HV et al. (1995) A 30-month study investigating the effect of adding triclosan/copolymer to a fluoride dentifrice. *Caries Res* **29**, 163–167.

Health Education Authority (HEA) (1994) *Health and Lifestyles: Black and Minority Ethnic Groups in England*. Health Education Authority, London.

HEA (1996) *The Scientific Basis of Dental Health Education* (ed R Levine). Health Education Authority, London.

Heath MR (1971) Dietary selection of elderly persons related to dental state. *Brit Dent J* **132**, 145–148.

Heft MW, McNeal DR, Knapp N, Jones J, Kincheloe J (1987) Carious missing and filled teeth among elderly in Florida. *J Dent Res* **66**, 185.

Hemmens ES, Blayney JR, Bradel SF, Harrison RW (1946) The microbic flora of the dental palque in relation to the beginning of caries. *J Dent Res* **25**, 195–205.

Hindle I, Downer MC, Speight PM (1996) Oral cancer in England and Wales 1901–1990. *Brit J Oral Maxillofacial Surg* **34**, 471–476.

Hinds K, Gregory JR (1995) *National Diet and Nutrition Survey: Children Aged $1\frac{1}{2}$ to $4\frac{1}{2}$ Years*, Vol. 2: *Report of the Dental Survey*. HMSO, London.

Hobson P (1980) The treatment of medically handicapped children. *Int Dent J* **30**, 6–13.

Hodges RE, Hood J, Canham J E, Sauberlich HE, Baker EM (1971) Clinical manifestations of ascorbic acid deficiency in man. *Am J Clin Nutr* **24**, 432–443.

Hogan J (1995) Dental Health. In *Community Child Health and Paediatrics* (eds Harvey, Miles, Smyth). Butterworth-Heineman, Oxford.

Holloway PJ, Shaw JH, Sweeney EA (1961) Effects of various surcose casein ratios in purfield diets on the teeth and supporting structures of rats. *Arch Oral Biol* **3**, 185–200.

Holloway PJ, Ellwood RP (1997) The prevalence,

causes and cosmetic importance of dental fluorosis in the United Kingdom: A review. *Commun Dent Health* **14**, 148–155

Holm-Pedersen P, Agerbaek N, Theilade E (1975) Experimental gingivitis in young and elderly individuals. *J Clin Periodontol* **2**, 14–24.

Holt RD (1991) Food and drinks at four daily time intervals in a group of young children. *Brit Dent J* **170**, 137–143.

Holt RD, Joels D, Bulman J, Maddick IH (1988) A third study of caries in pre-school aged children in Camden. *Brit Dent J* **165**, 87–91.

Holt RD, Morris CE, Winter GB, Downer MC (1994) Enamel opacities and dental caries in children who used a low fluoride toothpaste between 2 and 5 years of age. *Int Dent J* **44**, 331–341.

Hood J, Burns CA, Hodges RE (1970) Sjögren's syndrome in scurvy. *New Engl J Med* **282**, 1120–1124.

Horowitz SH, Driscoll WS, Meyers RJ *et al.* (1984) A new method for assessing the prevalence of dental fluorosis—the Tooth Surface Index of Fluorosis. *J Am Dent Assoc* **109**, 37–41.

Houwink B, Wagg BJ (1979) Effect of fluoride dentifrice usage during infancy upon enamel mottling of the permanent teeth. *Caries Res* **13**, 231–237.

Hussein I, Pollard MA, Curzon MEJ (1996) A comparison of the effects of some extrinsic and intrinsic sugars on dental plaque pH. *Int J Paediat Dent* **6**, 81–86.

Ikeda T, Sandham HJ, Bradley EL Jr. (1973) Changes in *Streptococcus mutans* and lactobacillus in plaque in relation to the initiation of dental caries in Negro children. *Arch Oral Biol* **18**, 555–566.

Imfeld T (1983) Acidogenic and erosive potential of soft drinks and mineral waters. In *Monographs in Oral Science*, Vol. 11: *Identification of Cow Caries Risk Dietary Components*. Karger, Basel, Switzerland, 165–174.

Imfeld T (1993) Efficacy of sweeteners and sugar substitutes in caries prevention. *Caries Res* **27**, S50-S55.

Imfeld T (1996) Dental erosion. Definition, classification and links. *Eur J Oral Sci* **104**, 151–155.

Imfeld T, Schmid R, Lutz F, Guggenheim B (1991) Cariogenicity of Milchschnitte (Ferrero GmbH) and apples in program-fed rats. *Caries Res* **25**, 352–358.

Infante PF, Gillespie GM (1974) An epidemiological study of linear enamel hypoplasia of deciduous anterior teeth in Guatemalan children. *Arch Oral Biol* **19**, 1055–1061.

Infante PF, Gillespie GM (1977) Enamel hypoplasia in relation to caries in Guatemalan children. *J Dent Res* **56**, 493–498.

International Agency for Research on Cancer (1985) Tobacco habits other than smoking; betel quid and areca-nut chewing and some related nitrosamines. *Monographs on the Evaluation of Carcinogenic Risk of Chemicals to Humans*. IARC Monograph No. 37, International Agency for Research on Cancer, Lyon, 141–200.

International Agency for Research on Cancer (1988) Alcohol Drinking. *Monographs on the Evaluation of the Carcinogenic Risk of Chemicals to Humans*. IARC Monograph No. 44, IARC, Lyon.

Ismail AI, Burt BA, Brunelle JA (1990) Oral health status of Mexican-Americans with low and high acculturation status. *J Public Health Dent* **50**, 24–31.

Jacobs A (1960) The buccal mucosa in anaemia. *J Clin Pathol* **13**, 463–468.

James WPT, Nelson M, Ralph A, Leather S (1997) The contribution of nutrition to inequalities in health. *Brit Med J* **314**, 1545–1549

Järvinen VK, Meurman JH, Hyvärinen H *et al.* (1988) Dental erosion and upper gastrointestinal disorders. *Oral Surg* **65**, 298–303.

Järvinen VK, Rytömaa II, Heinonen OP (1991) Risk factors in dental erosion. *J Dent Res* **70**, 942–947.

Jenkins GN (1983) Molybdenum. In *Trace Elements and Dental Disease* (eds MEJ Curzon, TE Cutress). John Wright, Boston.

Jenkins WMM, MacFarlane TW, Ferguson MM, Mason DK (1977) Nutritional deficiency in oral candidosis. *Int J Oral Surg* **6**, 204–210.

Johnsen D, Krejci C, Hack M, Fanaroff A (1984) Distribution of enamel defects and the association with respiratory distress in very low birth weight infants. *J Dent Res* **63**, 59–64.

Johnson JL, Moore LV, Kaneko B, Moore WE (1990) *Actinomyces georgiae* sp. nov., *Actinomyces gerencseriae* sp. nov., designation of two genospecies of *Actinomyces naeslundii*, and inclusion of *A. naeslundii* serotypes II and III and *Actinomyces viscosus* serotype II in *A. naeslundii* genospecies 2. *Int J Syst Bacteriol* **40**, 273–286.

Johnson IT, Southgate DAT, Durnin JVGA (1996) Intrinsic and non-milk sugars: does the distinction have analytical or physiological validity? *Int J Food Science and Nutr* **47**, 131–140.

Johnson NW, Warnakulasuriya KAAS (1993) Epidemiology and aetiology of oral cancer in the United Kingdom. *Commun Dent Health* **10**s, 13–29.

Jones RF (1961) The Paterson-Brown-Kelly syndrome, its relationship to iron deficiency and post-cricoid carcinoma. *J Laryngol* **75**, 529–543.

Jones S, Hussey R, Lennon MA (1996) Dental health related behaviours in low and high caries areas in St Helens, North West England. *Brit Dent J* **181**, 13–17.

Jones CM, Taylor GO, Whittle JG, Evans IO, Trotter DP (1997). Water fluoridation, tooth decay in 5 year olds, and social deprivation measured by the Jarman score: analysis of data from British dental surveys. *Brit Med J* **315**, 514–517.

Kato I, Nomura AMY, Stemmerman GN, Chyon PM (1992) Prospective study of the association of alcohol with cancer of the upper aerodigestive tract and other sites. *Canc Causes Cont* **3**, 145–151.

Kawamura Y, Hou XG, Sultana F, Liu S, Yamamoto H, Ezaki T (1995) Transfer of *Streptococcus adjacens* and *Streptococcus defectivus* to *Abiotrophia* gen. nov. as *Abiotrophia adiacens* comb. nov. and *Abiotrophia defectiva* comb. nov., respectively. *Int J Syst Bacteriol* **45**, 798–803.

Käyser AF (1981). Shortened dental arches and oral function. *J Oral Rehab* **8**, 457–462.

Keller AZ, Terris M (1965) The association of alcohol and tobacco with cancer of the mouth and pharynx. *Am J Publ Health* **55**, 1578–1585.

Kelly AB (1919) Spasm at entrance to the oesophagus. *J Laryngol* **34**, 285–289.

Khaw KT, Woodhouse P (1995) Interrelation of vitamin C, infection, haemostatic factors, and cardiovascular disease *Brit Med J* **310**, 1559–1563.

Kilian M, Mikkelson L, Henricsen J (1989) Taxonomic study of viridans streptococci: description of *Streptococcus gordonii* sp. nov. and amended descriptions of *Streptococcus sanguis* (White and Niven, 1946), *Streptococcus oralis* (Bridge and Sneath, 1982) and *Streptococcus mitis* (Andrews and Horder, 1906). *Int J Syst Bacteriol* **39**, 471–484.

Kinirons MJ (1989) Dental health of patients suffering from cystic fibrosis in Northern Ireland. *Commun Dent Health* **6**, 113–120.

Kiyak HA (1993) Age and culture: influence on oral health behaviour. *Int Dent J* **43**, 9–16.

Klatsky AL, Friedman GD, Sigelaub AB (1981) Alcohol and mortality. A ten-year Kaiser-Permanente experience. *Ann Int Med* **95**, 139–145.

Kleinman DV, Drury TF (1996) Oral health in the United States, 1988–1991: the first three years of the Third National Health and Nutrition Examination Survey. *J Dent Res* **75**, 617.

Kleinman DV, Swango PA, Niessen LC (1991) Epidemiologic studies of oral mucosal conditions—methodologic issues. *Comm Dent Oral Epidemiol* **19**, 129–140.

Ko YC, Chiang TA, Chiang SJ, Hsieh SF (1992) Prevalence of betel quid chewing habit in Taiwan and related sociodemographic factors. *J Oral Pathol Med* **21**, 261–264.

Kohler B, Andreen I, Jonsson B (1984) The effect of caries preventive measures in mothers on dental caries and the oral presence of the bacteria *Streptococcus mutans* and lactobacilli in their children. *Arch Oral Biol* **29**, 879–883.

Kohler B, Andreen I (1994) Influence of caries preventive measures in mothers on cariogenic bacteria and caries experience in their children. *Arch Oral Biol* **39**, 907–911.

Könönen E, Asikainen S, Jousimies Somer H (1992) The early colonization of gram negative anaerobic bacteria in edentulous infants. *Oral Microbiol Immunol* **7**, 28–31.

Kristofferson K, Birkhed D (1987) Effects of partial sugar restriction for 6 weeks on numbers of *Streptococcus mutans* in saliva and interdental plaque in man. *Caries Res* **21**, 79–86.

Kulasegaram R, Downer MC, Jullien JA *et al.* (1995) Case-control study of oral dysplasia and risk habits among patients of a dental hospital. *Eur J Canc* **31B**, 227–231.

La Vecchia C, Franceschi S, Levi F *et al.* (1993). Diet and human oral carcinoma in Europe. *Eur J Canc* **29B**, 17–22.

La Vecchia C, Negri E, D'Avanzo B *et al.* (1991). Dietary indicators of oral and pharyngeal cancer. *Int J Epidemiol* **20**, 39–44.

Lamey P, Hammond A, Allan BF, McIntosh WB (1986) Vitamin status of patients with burning mouth syndrome and the response to replacement therapy. *Brit Dent J* **160**, 81–83.

Lappalainen R, Nyyssonen V (1987) Self-assessed chewing ability of Finnish adults with removable dentures. *Gerodontology* **3**, 238–241.

Larsson LG, Sandstrom A, Westling P (1975) Relationship of Plummer-Vinson disease to cancer of the upper alimentary tract in Sweden. *Cancer Res* **35**, 3308–3316.

Leininger MM (1988) Leininger's theory of nursing: cultural care diversity and university. *Nursing Sci Quart* **1**, 152–160.

Levine RS, Keen JH (1974) Neonatal enamel hypoplasia in association with symptomatic neonatal hypocalcemia. *Brit Dent J* **137**, 429–433.

Levine MJ, Reddy MS, Tabak LA *et al.* (1987) Structural aspects of salivary glycoproteins. *J Dent Res* **66**, 436–441.

Lewis MA, MacFarlane TW, McGowan DA, MacDonald DG (1988) Assessment of the pathogenicity of bacterial species isolated from acute dentoalveolar abscesses. *J Med Microbiol* **27**, 109–116.

Li Y, Caufield PW (1995) The fidelity of initial acquisition of mutans streptococci by infants from their mothers. *J Dent Res* **74**, 681–685.

Li Y, Navia JM, Bian JY (1996) Caries experience in deciduous dentition of rural Chinese children 3–5 years old in relation to the presence or absence of enamel hypoplasia. *Caries Res* **30**, 8–15.

Linkosalo E, Markkonam H (1985) Dental erosion in relation to lactovegetarian diet. *Scand J Dent Res* **93**, 436–441.

Lippman SM, Batsakis JG, Toth BB *et al.* (1993) Comparison of low dose isoretinoin with beta-carotene to prevent oral carcinogenesis. *New Engl J Med* **328**, 15–20.

Lippman SM, Lee JS, Lotan R, Hong WK (1990) Chemoprevention of upper aerodigestive tract cancers: a report of the third upper aerodigestive cancer task force workshop. *Head and Neck* **12**, 5–20.

Löe H, Ancrud A, Boysen H, Smith M (1978) The natural history of periodontal disease in man. *J Periodontol* **49**, 607–620.

Loesche WJ, Grossman NS, Earnest R, Corpron R (1984) The effect of chewing xylitol gum on the plaque and saliva levels of *Streptococcus mutans*. *J Am Dent Assoc* **108**, 587–592.

Loesche WJ, Straffon LH (1979) Longitudinal investigation of the role of *Streptococcus mutans* in human fissure decay. *Infection and Immunity* **26**, 498–507.

Lord Jauncey (1983) *Opinion of Lord Jauncey: Mrs Catherine McColl v Strathclyde Regional Council*. Court of Session, Edinburgh.

Lucas VS, Beighton D, Roberts GJ, Challacombe SJ (1997) Changes in the oral streptococcal flora of children undergoing allogenic bone marrow transplantation. *J Infect* **35**, 135–141.

Lunt RC, Law DB (1974) A review of the chronology of calcification of deciduous teeth. *J Am Dent Assoc* **89**, 599–606.

Lussi A, Scaffner M, Hotz P, Suter P (1991) Dental

erosion in a population of Swiss adults. *Comm Dent Oral Epidemiol* **19**, 286–290.

Macfarlane GJ (1993) *The Epidemiology of Oral Cancer*. Thesis, University of Bristol.

Macfarlane GJ, Boyle P, Scully C (1992) Oral cancer in Scotland: changing incidence and mortality. *Brit Med J* **305**, 1121–1123.

Mahmood ZSH, Jafarey NA, Aijaz AS (1974) Cancer trends in Karachi. *J Pakistan Med Assoc* **24**, 87–93.

Mäkinen KK (1989) Latest dental studies on xylitol and mechanism of action of xylitol in caries limitation. In *Progress in Sweeteners* (ed T Grenby). Elsevier, London, 331–362.

Mäkinen KK, Bennett CA, Hujoel PP *et al.* (1995) Xylitol chewing gums and caries rates: a 40-month cohort study. *J Dent Res* **74**, 1904–1913.

Mäkinen KK, Soderling E, Isokangas P, Tenovuo J, Tiekso J (1989) Oral biochemical status and depression of *Streptococcus mutans* in children during 24 to 36 month use of xylitol chewing gum. *Caries Res* **23**, 261–267.

Manning RH, Edgar WM (1992) Intra oral models for studying de- and re-mineralisation in man: methodology and measurement. *J Dent Res* **71**, 895–900.

Manson JD, Eley BM (1995) *Outline of Periodontics*, 3rd edn. Butterworth-Heinemann, Oxford.

Marques APF, Messer LB (1992) Nutrient intake and dental caries in the primary dentition. *Pediat Dent* **14**, 314–321.

Marsh PD, Martin M (1992) *Oral Microbiology*, 3rd edn. Chapman and Hall, London.

Marsh PD, Percival RS, Challacombe SJ (1992) The influence of denture wearing and age on the oral microflora. *J Dent Res* **71**, 1374–1381.

Marshall JR, Graham S, Haughey BP, *et al.* (1992) Smoking, alcohol, dentition and diet in the epidemiology of oral cancer. *Eur J Canc* **28B**, 9–15.

Marthaler TM (1967) Epidemiological and clinical dental findings in relation to intake of carbohydrates. *Caries Res* **1**, 222–238.

Marthaler TM (1983) Practical aspects of fluoridation. *Helvetica Odontologiska Acta* **27**, 39–56.

Mashberg A, Boffeta P, Winkelman R, Garfinkel L (1993) Tobacco smoking, alcohol drinking and cancer of the oral cavity and oropharynx among US veterans. *Cancer* **72**, 1369–1375.

Matee MIN, van't Hof MA, Maselle SY, Mitx FHM. (1994) Nursing caries, linear hypoplasia, and nursing and weaning habits in Tanzanian infants. *Comm Dent Oral Epidemiol* **22**, 289–293.

Mathur M, Ramalingaswami V, Deo MG (1972) Influence of protein deficiency on 19S antibody-forming cells in rats and mice. *J Nutr* **102**, 841–846.

Mayhall JT (1975) Canadian Inuit caries experience 1969–1973. *J Dent Res* **54**, 1245.

McDonald SP, Cowell CR, Sheiham A (1981) Methods of preventing dental caries used by dentists on their own children. *Brit Dent J* **151**, 118–121.

McLaughlin JK, Gridley G, Block G *et al.* (1988) Dietary factors in oral and pharyngeal cancer. *J Nat Canc Inst* **80**, 1237–1243.

Meechan JG, Welbury RR (1996) Medical problems affecting the management of children in dentistry. *Dental Update* **23**, 242–245.

Mellanby M (1918) An experimental study of the influence of diet on teeth formation. *Lancet* **ii**, 767–770.

Mellanby M, Martin WJ (1962) Dental structure and disease in some 5-year-old Indian children compared with the same age-group in London. *Arch Oral Biol* **7**, 633–650.

Mellander M, Norén JG, Fredén H, Kjellmer I (1982) Mineralization defects in deciduous teeth of low birth weight infants. *Acta Paediatrica Scandanivia* **71**, 727–733.

Menaker L, Navia JM (1973) Effect of undernutrition during the perinatal period on caries development in the rat. III effect of undernutrition on biochemical parameters in the developing mandibular salivary gland. *J Dent Res* **52**, 688–691.

Merletti F, Boffetta P, Ferro G *et al.* (1991) Occupation and cancer of the oral cavity or oropharynx in Turin, Italy. *Scand J Work Environ Health* **17**, 248–254.

Merletti F, Boffetta P, Ciccone G, *et al.* (1989) Role of tobacco and alcoholic beverages in the etiology of cancer of the oral cavity/oropharynx in Torino, Italy. *Canc Res* **49**, 4919–4924.

Meyers HM (1978) *Fluorides and Dental Fluorosis. Monographs in Oral Science*, No. 7. Karger, Basel.

Midda M, Konig KG (1994) Report of an FDI Working Group: Nutrition, diet and oral health. *Int Dent J* **44**, 599–612.

Millward A, Shaw L, Smith AJ, Rippin JW, Harrington E (1994a) The distribution and severity of tooth wear and the relationship between erosion and dietary constituents in a group of children. *Int J Paediat Dent* **4**, 152–157.

Millward A, Shaw L, Smith A (1994b) Dental erosion in four-year-old children from differing socio-economic backgrounds. *J Dent Child* **61**, 262–266.

Milnes A R (1996) Description and epidemiology of nursing caries. *J Public Health Dent* **56**, 38–50.

Milnes AR, Bowden GH (1985) The micoflora associated with devloping lesions of nursing caries. *Caries Res* **19**, 289–297.

Milosevic A, Young PI, Lennon MA (1993) The prevalence of tooth wear in 14-year-old school children in Liverpool. *Commun Dent Health* **11**, 83–86.

Milsom K, Mitropoulos CM (1990) Enamel defects in 8-year-old children in fluoridated and non-fluoridated parts of Cheshire. *Caries Res* **24**, 286–289.

Ministry of Agriculture, Food and Fisheries (1997) *National Food Survey 1996*. HMSO, London.

Mitchell K, Ferguson MM, Lucie NP, MacDonald DG (1986) Epithelial dysplasia in the oral mucosa associated with pernicious anaemia. *Brit Dent J* **161**, 259–260.

Mitropoulos CM, Langford JW, Robinson DJ (1988) Differences in dental caries experience in 14-year-old children in fluoridated South Birmingham and in Bolton in 1987. *Brit Dent J* **164**, 349–350.

Moller (1851) Klinische Bermerkungen uber einige weniger bekannte Krankheiten der Zunge. *Deutsche Klinik* **3**, 273–275.

Møller, H (1989). Changing incidence of cancer of the

tongue, oral cavity and pharynx in Denmark. *J Oral Pathol Med* **18**, 224–229.

Monson RR, Lyon JL (1975). Proportional mortality among alcoholics. *Cancer* **36**, 1077–1079.

Moore WJ, Corbett ME (1978) Dental caries experience in man: historical, anthropological and cultural diet-caries relationships. The English experience. In *Diet, Nutrition and Dental Caries* (ed NH Rowe). University of Michigan School of Dentistry, 3–19.

Moore WE, Moore LH, Ranney RR, Smibert RM, Burmeister JA, Schenkein HA (1991) The microflora of periodontal sites showing active destructive progression. *J Clin Periodontol* **18**, 729–739.

Moore LM, Nielsen CR and Mistretta CM (1982) Sucrose taste thresholds: age-related differences. *J Gerontol* **37**, 64–69.

Morley JE (1986) Nutritional status of the elderly. *Am J Med* **81**, 565–570.

Moynihan PJ (1995) The relationship between diet, nutrition and dental health: an overview and update for the 1990s. *Nutr Res Rev* **8**, 193–224.

Moynihan PJ, Holt RD (1996) The national diet and nutrition survey of 1.5 to 4.5 year old children: summary of the findings of the dental survey. *Brit Dent J* **181**, 328–332.

Moynihan PJ, Snow S, Jepson NJ, Butler TJ (1994) Intake of non-starch polysaccharide (dietary fibre) in edentulous and dentate persons: an observational study. *Brit Dent J* **177**, 243–247.

Moynihan PJ, Wright WG, Walton AG (1996) A comparison of the relative acidogenic potential of infant milk and soya infant formula: a plaque pH study. *Int J Paediat Dent* **6**, 177–181.

Mr Justice Kenny (1963). *Fluoridation. Judgement delivered by Mr Justice Kenny in the High Court, Dublin*. Department of Health, Dublin.

Murrah VA (1985) Diabetes mellitus and associated oral manifestations: a review. *J Oral Pathol* **14**, 271–281.

Murray JJ (ed) (1986) *Appropriate Use of Fluorides for Human Health*. World Health Organisation, Geneva.

Murray JJ (ed) (1990) *The Prevention of Dental Disease*, 2nd edn. Oxford University Press, New York, 34–43.

Murray JJ, Rugg-Gunn AJ, Jenkins GN. *Fluoride in Caries Prevention*, 3rd edn. Butterworth-Heinemann, Oxford.

Murray JJ, Shaw L (1979) Classification and prevalence of enamel opacities in the human deciduous and permanent dentition. *Arch Oral Biol* **24**, 7–13.

Murti PR, Gupta PC, Bhonsle RB, Daftary DK, Mehta FS, Pindborg JJ (1992) Smokeless tobacco use in India: effects on oral mucosa. Smoking and Tobacco Control Monograph 2. *NIH Publication* **3461**, 51–65.

Naccache H, Simard PL, Trahan L *et al.* (1992) Factors affecting the ingestion of fluoride dentifrice by children. *J Public Health Dent* **52**, 222–226.

Nanda Sanjit, Nanda Smiti, Tewari AD *et al.* (1984) Calcium metabolism in marasmus. *Indian Pediat* **21**, 891–895.

Narhi TO, Meurman JH, Ainamo A *et al.* (1992). Association between salivary flow rate and the use of systematic medication among 76-, 81-, and 86-year-old inhabitants in Helsinki, Finland. *J Dent Res* **71**, 1875–1880.

National Food Alliance (1995). *Easy to Swallow, Hard to Stomach*. The National Food Alliance, London.

Naylor MN, Murray JJ (1989) Fluorides and dental caries. In *The Prevention of Dental Disease* (ed JJ Murray). Oxford University Press, Oxford.

Needleman HL, Allred E, Bellinger D, Leviton A, Rabinowitz M, Iverson K (1992) Antedecents and correlates of hypoplastic enamel defects of primary incisors. *Pediat Dent* **14**, 158–166.

Nelson M (1993) Nutritional content of children's diets and the health implications. In *Food for Children Influencing Choice and Investing in Health*. National Forum for Coronary Heart Disease Prevention, London.

Ness AR, Khaw KT, Bingham S, Day NE (1996a) Vitamin C status and respiratory function. *Eur J Clin Nutr* **50**, 573–579.

Ness AR, Khaw KT, Bingham S, Day NE (1996b) Vitamin C status and undiagnosed angina. *J Cardiovasc Risk* **3**, 373–377.

Ness AR, Powles JW, Khaw KT (1996c) Vitamin C and cardiovascular disease. *J Cardiovasc Risk* **3**, 513–521.

Newbrun E, Hoover C, Mettraux G, Graf H (1980) Comparison of dietary habits and dental health of subjects with hereditary fructose intolerance and control subjects. *J Am Dent Assoc* **101**, 619–626.

Newton JP, Yemm R, Abel RW, Menhinick S (1993) Changes in human jaw muscles with age and dental state. *Gerodontology* **10**, 16–22.

Nikiforuk G, Fraser D (1981) The aetiology of enamel hypoplasia; a unifying concept. *J Pediat* **98**, 888–893.

Noorda WD, Purdell Lewis DJ, van Montfort AM, Weerkamp AH (1988) Monobacterial and mixed bacterial plaques of *Streptococcus mutans* and *Veillonella alcalescens* in an artificial mouth: development, metabolism, and effect on human dental enamel. *Caries Res* **22**, 342–347.

North Western Regional Health Authority (NWRHA) (1994). *Paediatric Dental Anaesthesia Rates 89–93*. Department of Dental Public Health, North Western Regional Health Authority.

Nunn JH (1996) Prevalence of dental erosion and the implications for oral health. *J Oral Sci* **104**, 156–161.

Nunn JH (1997) Childhood disability. In *Paediatric Dentistry* (ed RR Welbury). Oxford University Press, Oxford, 375–394.

Nylen MV (1964) Electron microscope and allied biophysical approaches to the study of enamel mineralisation. *J Microscopy Soc* **83**, 135–141.

Nyvad B, Fejerskov O (1985) Active root surface caries converted into inactive caries as a response to oral hygiene. *Scand J Dent Res* **94**, 281–284.

O'Brien M (1994) *Children's Dental Health in the United Kingdom 1993*. Office of Population Censuses and Surveys, London.

Odds FC, Bernaerts R (1994) CHROMagar Candida, a new differential isolation medium for presumptive identification of clinically important *Candida* species. *J Clin Microbiol* **32**, 1923–1929.

Office of Population Censuses and Surveys (OPCS) (1980). *Classification of Occupations*. HMSO, London.

OPCS (1992) *County Monitors*. OPCS, London.

OPCS (1994) *Cancer Statistics Registrations*. Series MB1, No. 21, HMSO, London.

Oho T, Rahemtulla F, Mansson Rahemtulla B, Hjerpe A (1992) Purification and characterization of a glycosylated proline rich protein from human parotid saliva. *Int J Biochem* **24**, 1159–1168.

Olojugba OO, Lennon MA (1987) Dental caries experience in 5- and 12-year old school children in Ondo State, Nigeria in 1977 and 1983. *Commun Dent Health* **4**, 129–135.

Olojugba OO, Lennon MA (1990) Sugar consumption in 5- and 12-year old school children in Ondo State, Nigeria in 1985. *Commun Dent Health* **7**, 259–265.

Oosterhaven SP, Westert GP, Schaub RMH, van der Bilt A (1988) Social and psychologic implications of missing teeth for chewing ability. *Comm Dent Oral Epidemiol* **16**, 79–82.

Osborn JW (ed.) (1981) *Dental Anatomy and Embryology*. Blackwell Scientific Publications, Oxford.

Österberg T, Steen B (1982) Relationship between dental state and dietary intake in 70-year-old males and females in Gothenberg, Sweden: A population study. *J Oral Rehab* **9**, 509–521.

Owen RD (1950) The problem of hypopharyngeal carcinoma. *Proc Roy Soc Med* **43**, 157–170.

Owen D (1996) Size, structure and growth of the ethnic minority population. In *Ethnicity in the 1991 Census* Vol. 1 (eds D Coleman, J Salt). HMSO, London.

Pack ARC (1984) Folate mouthwash: effects on established gingivitis in periodontal patients. *J Clin periodontol* **1**, 619–628.

Pacy PJ (1989) Nutrition patterns and deficiencies. In *Ethnic Factors in Health and Disease* (eds JK Cruickshank, DG Beevers). Wright, London.

Papas AS, Joshi A, Palmer CA, Giunta JL, Dwyer JT (1995) Relationship of diet to root caries. *Am J Clin Nutr* **61**, S423–S429.

Parkin DM, Muir CS (1992) Comparability and quality of data. In *Cancer Incidence in Five Continents*, Vol. VI (eds DM Parkin, CS Muir, SL Whelan). IARC Scientific Publications, No. 120. International Agency for Research on Cancer, Lyon, 45–55.

Parkin DM, Pisani P, Ferlay J (1993) Estimates of the worldwide incidence of eighteen major cancers in 1985. *Int J Canc* **54**, 594–606.

Paster BJ, Dewhirst FE, Olsen I, Fraser GJ (1994) Phylogeny of *Bacteroides*, *Prevotella*, and *Porphyromonas* spp. and related bacteria. *J Bacteriol* **176**, 725–732.

Pearce C, Bowden GH, Evans M *et al.* (1995) Identification of pioneer viridans streptococci in the oral cavity of human neonates. *J Med Microbiol* **42**, 67–72.

Paterson DR (1919) A clinical type of dysphagia. *J Laryngol, Rhinol Otol* **34**, 289–291.

Pearson M (1991) Ethnic differences in infant health. *Arch Diseases Childh* **66**, 88–90.

Pearson NK (1994) Oral health status and dental treatment needs of an adult Bangladeshi population resident in Tower Hamlets. MSc Thesis, University of London.

Pendrys DG, Stamm JW (1990) Relationship of total fluoride intake to beneficial effects and enamel fluorosis. *J Dent Res* **69**, S529–S538.

Perry JL, Miller GR (1987) Umbelliferyl labeled galactosaminide as an aid in the identification of *Candida albicans*. *J Clin Microbiol* **25**, 2424–2425.

Petersen PE (1983) Dental health among workers at a Danish chocolate factory. *Comm Dent Oral Epidemiol* **11**, 37–341.

Pike D C (1994) Manufacture and marketing of sugar free confectionery. In *Sugarless—Towards the Year 2000* (ed RJ Rugg-Gunn). Royal Society of Chemistry, London, 136–146.

Pindborg JJ (1982) Aetiology of developmental enamel defects not related to fluorosis. *Int Dent J* **32**, 123–134.

Pitts NB, Palmer JD (1994) The dental caries experience of 5-, 12- and 14-year-old children in Great Britain. Surveys coordinated by the British Association for the Study of Community Dentistry in 1990–1993. *Commun Dent Health* **11**, 42–52.

Pitts NB (1997) Do we understand which children need and get appropriate dental care? *Brit Dent J* **182**, 273–278.

Platz H, Fries R, Hudec M (1986) Prognoses of oral cavity carcinomas. Results of a multi-centre retrospective observational study. Hanser, München.

Pollard MA (1996) Potential cariogenicity of starches and fruits as assessed by the plaque sampling method and an intraoral cariogenicity test. *Caries Res* **29**, 68–74.

Pollard MA, Imfeld T, Higham SM *et al.* (1996) Acidogenic potential and total salivary carbohydrate content of expectorants following the consumption of some cereal based foods and fruits. *Caries Res* **30**, 132–137.

Prendergast MJ, Beal JF, Williams SA (1993) An investigation of non-response bias by comparison of dental health in 5 year old children according to parental response to a questionnaire. *Commun Dent Health* **10**, 225–234.

Primosch RE (1980) Tetracycline discoloration, enamel defects and dental caries in patients with cystic fibrosis. *Oral Surg* **50**, 503–508.

Purvis RJ, Barrie WJM, Mackay GS, *et al.* (1973) Enamel hypoplasia of the teeth associated with neonatal tetany: manifestation of maternal vitamin deficiency. *Lancet* **ii**, 811–814.

Ramirez M (1980) Recognising and understanding diversity: multiculturalism and the Chicano movement in psychology. In *Chicano Psychology*, 2nd edn (eds JL Martinez, RH Mendoza). Academic Press, New York.

Rasmussen P, Espelid I (1980) Coeliac disease and dental malformation. *J Dent Health Childh* **47**, 424.

Ratcliffe P (1996) Social geography and ethnicity: a theoretical conceptual and substantive overview. In *Ethnicity in the 1991 Census*, Vol. 3. HMSO, London.

Rauch S, Gorlin RJ (1970) Diseases of the Salivary Glands. In *Oral Pathology* (eds RJ Gorlin, HM Goldman). Mosby, St Louis, 994.

Reece JA, Swallow JN (1970) Carrots and dental health. *Brit Dent J* **128**, 535–539.

Rees P, Phillips D (1996) Geographical spread—a national picture. In *Ethnicity in the 1991 Census*, Vol. 3. HMSO, London.

Reichart PA, Ulrich M, Sampan S, Heinz G, Kangwanpong T (1987) Precancerous and other oral mucosal lesions related to chewing, smoking and drinking habits in Thailand. *Comm Dent Oral Epidemiol* **15**, 152–160.

Rennie JS, MacDonald DG, Dagg JH (1984) Iron and the oral epithelium: a review. *J Roy Soc Med* **77**, 602–607.

Reynolds EC, Black CL (1987) Confectionery composition and rat caries. *Caries Res* **21**, 538–545.

Rich AM, Radden BG (1984) Squamous cell carcinoma of the oral mucosa: a review of 244 cases in Australia. *J Oral Pathol* **13**, 459–471.

Riordan PJ (1993) Fluoride supplements in caries prevention: a literature review and proposal for a new dosage schedule. *J Public Health Dent* **53**, 174–189.

Robb ND, Cruwys E, Smith BGN (1991) Regurgitation erosion as a possible cause of tooth wear in ancient British populations. *Arch Oral Biol* **36**, 595–602.

Robb N, Smith B, Geidrys-Leeper E (1995) The distribution of erosion in the dentitions of patients with eating disorders. *Brit Dent J* **178**, 171–175.

Roberts GJ (1982) Is breast feeding a possible cause of dental caries? *J Dentistry* 10, 545–551.

Roberts IF, Roberts GJ (1979) Relations between medicines sweetened with sucrose and dental disease. *Brit Med J* **ii**, 14–16.

Rock WP (1994) Young children and fluoride toothpaste. *Brit Dent J* **177**, 17–20.

Rock WP, Sabieha AM (1997) The relationship between reported toothpaste usage in infancy and fluorosis of permanent incisors. *Brit Dent J* **183**, 165–170.

Rose JA (1968) Aetiology of angular cheilosis. Iron metabolism. *Brit Dent J* **152**, 67–72.

Rose JA (1971) Folic acid deficiency as a cause of angular cheilitis. *Lancet* **ii**, 453–454.

Rosen EU, Geefhuysin J (1971) Immunoglobulin levels in protein calorie malnutrition. *South African J Med*, 980–982.

Rothman K, Keller A (1972) The effect of joint exposure to alcohol and tobacco on the risk of cancer of the mouth and pharynx. *J Chron Disease* **25**, 711–716.

Royal College of Physicians (1976) *Fluoride Teeth and Health*. RCP, London.

Royal Pharmaceutical Society of Great Britain/British Medical Association (1996) *British National Formulary*. RPSGB, London.

Rudat K (1994) Health and lifestyles. In *Black and Minority Ethnic Groups in England*. The Health Education Authority, London.

Rugg-Gunn AJ (1989) Lycasin and the prevention of dental caries. In *Progress in Sweeteners* (ed T Grenby). Elsevier, London, 311–329.

Rugg-Gunn AJ (1993a) *Nutrition and Dental Health*. Oxford University Press, Oxford.

Rugg-Gunn AJ (1993b) Nutrition, diet and dental public health. *Commun Dent Health* **10**, S47–S56.

Rugg-Gunn AJ, Carmichael CL, Ferrell RS (1988) Effect of fluoridation and secular trends in caries in 5-year-old children living in Newcastle and Northumberland. *Brit Dent J* **165**, 359–364.

Rugg-Gunn AJ, Cottrell RC (1997) Debating Nutrition. Is the concept of non-milk extrinsic sugars valid? *Brit Nutr Bull* **22**, 47–55.

Rugg-Gunn AJ, Edgar WM, Geddes DAM, Jenkins GN (1975) The effect of different meal patterns upon plaque pH in human subjects. *Brit Dent J* **139**, 351–356.

Rugg-Gunn AJ, Hackett AF, Appleton DR, Jenkins GN, Eastoe JE (1984) Relationship between dietary habits and caries increment assessed over two years in 405 adolescent schoolchildren. *Arch Oral Biol* **29**, 983–992.

Rugg-Gunn AJ, Hackett AF, Appleton DR, Moynihan PJ (1986) The dietary intake of added and natural sugars in 405 English adolescents. *Hum Nutr; Appl Nutr* **40A**, 115–124.

Rugg-Gunn AJ, Hackett AF, Appleton DR, Eastoe JE, Dowthwaite L, Wright WG (1987a) The water intake of 405 Northumbrian adolescents aged 12–14 years. *Brit Dent J* **162**, 335–340.

Rugg-Gunn AJ, Hackett AF, Appleton DR (1987b) Relative cariogenicity of starch and sugars in a two-year longitudinal study of 405 English schoolchildren. *Caries Res* **21**, 464–473.

Rugg-Gunn AJ, Roberts GJ, Wright WG (1985) The effect of human milk on plaque in situ and enamel dissolution in vitro compared with bovine milk, lactose and sucrose. *Caries Res* **19**, 327–334.

Russell AL (1963) International nutriton surveys; a summary of preliminary dental findings. *J Dent Res* **42**, 233–244.

Rustung E (1949) Studies on serum iron. *Acta Dermato-Venereologica* (*Stockholm*) **29**, 1–40.

Ryssel HJ, Brunner KW, Bollag,W (1971) Die orale Anwendung von Vitamin A-Säure bei Leukoplakien. Hyperkeratosen und Plattenepithel-karzinom: Ergebnisse und Verträglichkeit. *Schweizer Medizinische Wochenschrift* **101**, 1027–1030.

Sansone C, Van Houte J, Joshipura K, Kent R, Margolis HC (1993) The association of mutans streptococci and non mutans streptococci capable of acidogenesis at a low pH with dental caries on enamel and root surfaces. *J Dent Res* **72**, 508–516.

Sauberlich HE, Machlin LJ (1992) Beyond deficiency: new views on the function and health effects of vitamins. *Ann NY Acad Sci* **669**.

Scheifer KH, Ludwid W (1996) Phylogeny of the genus lactobacillus and related genera. *Syst Appl Microbiol* **18**, 461–467.

Scheinin A (1979) Influence of the diagnostic level on caries incidence in two controlled clinical trials. *Caries Res* **13**, 91.

Scheinin A, Makinen KK (1975) Turku sugar studies I-XXI. *Acta Odontologica Scandanavica* **33**s, 70.

Scheutzel P (1996) Etiology of dental erosion—intrinsic factors. *Eur J Oral Sci* **104**, 178–190.

Schieve JF, Rundles RW (1949) Response of lingual manifestations of pernicious anaemia to pteroylglutamic acid and vitamin B12. *Oral Surg, Oral Med, Oral Pathol* **2**, 1255–1263.

Schleifer KH, Ludwig W (1996) Phylogeny of the genus lactobacillus and related genera. *Syst Appl Microbiol* **18**, 461–467.

Schmidt W, Popham RE (1981) The role of drinking and smoking in mortality from cancer and other causes in male alcoholics. *Cancer* **47**, 1031–1041.

Schupbach P, Osterwalder V, Guggenheim B (1995) Human root caries: microbiota in plaque covering sound, carious and arrested carious root surfaces. *Caries Res* **29**, 382–395.

Scott J (1987) Structural age changes in salivary glands. In *The Aging Mouth*, Vol. 6 (ed DB Ferguson). Karger, Basle, 40–62.

Scott J, Baum BJ (1990) Oral effects of ageing. In *Oral Manifestations of Systemic Disease* (eds JH Jones, DK Mason). Baillière Tindall, London, 311–338.

Scott JH, Symons NBB (1982). *Introduction to Dental Anatomy*, 9th edn. Churchill Livingston, Edinburgh, 122.

Scott J, Valentine JA, St. Hill CA, Balasooriya BAW (1983) A quantitative histological analysis of the effects of age and sex on human lingual epithelium. *Journal de Biologie Buccale* **11**, 303–315.

Scully C (1989) The sore mouth (1–4) In *The Mouth and Perioral Tissues*, Vol. 2 (ed C Scully). Heineman, Oxford, 159–226.

Scully C, Boyle P (1992) Vitamin A related compounds in the chemoprevention of potentially malignant oral lesions and carcinoma. *Eur J Canc* **28B**, 87–90.

Scully C, Cawson RA (1993) *Medical Problems in Dentistry*, 3rd edn. Wright, Oxford, 197.

Senior PA, Bhopal R (1994) Ethnicity as a variable in epidemiological research. *Brit Med J* **309**, 327–330.

Seow WK, Latham SC (1986) The spectrum of dental manifestations in vitamin-D-resistant rickets and implications for management. *Pediat Dent* **8**, 245–250.

Seppa L, Pollanen L, Hausen (1988) *Streptococcus mutans* counts obtained by a dip-slide method in relation to caries frequency, sucrose intake and the flow rate of saliva. *Caries Res* **22**, 226–279.

Shammas MH, Benedict EB (1958) Oesophageal webs. A report of 58 cases and an attempt at classification. *New Engl J Med* **259**, 378–384.

Shaw L (1997) Medically compromised children. In *Paediatric Dentistry* (ed RR Welbury). Oxford University Press, Oxford, 354–371.

Shaw JH, Griffiths D (1963) Dental abnormalities in rats attributable to protein defiency during reproduction. *J Nutr* **80**, 123–141.

Shearer TR (1983) Selenium. In *Trace Elements and Dental Disease* (eds MEJ Curzon, TE Cutress), John Wright, Boston.

Sheiham A (1983) Sugars and dental decay. *Lancet* **i**, 282–284.

Sheiham A (1991) Why free sugar consumption should be below 15 kg per person per year in indus-trialised countries: the dental evidence. *Brit Dent J* **167**, 63–65.

Shklar G (1966) The effects of ageing upon oral mucosa. *J Invest Dermatol* **47**, 115–120.

Shklar G, Schwartz J (1993) Oral cancer inhibition by micronutrients. The experimental basis for clinical trials. *Eur J Canc* **29B**, 9–16.

Silva MF de A, Jenkins GN, Burgess RC, Sandham HJ (1986) Effects of cheese on experimental caries in human subjects. *Caries Res* **20**, 263–269.

Silver DH (1987) A longitudinal study of infant feeding practice, diet and caries, related to social class in children aged 3 and 7–10 years. *Brit Dent J* **163**, 296–300.

Silverman S, Bhargava K, Mani N *et al.* (1976) Malignant transformation and natural history of oral leukoplakia in 57,518 industrial workers in Gujarat, India. *Cancer* **38**, 1790–1795.

Silverman S, Renstrup G, Pindborg JJ (1963a) Studies in oral leukoplakias. III. Effects of vitamin A, comparing clinical, histopathologic, cytologic and hematologic responses. *Acta Odontologica Scandinavica* **21**, 271–292.

Silverman S, Renstrup G, Pindborg JJ (1963b) Studies on oral leukoplakias. VII. Further investigations on the effects of vitamin A on keratinization. *Acta Odontologica Scandinavica* **21**, 553–570.

Slack GL, Martin WJ (1958) Apples and dental health. *Brit Dent J* **105**, 366–371.

Slade EW, Bartuska D, Rose LF, Cohen DW (1976) Vitamin E and periodontal disease. *J Periodontol* **47**, 352–354.

Slots J, Listgarten MA (1988) *Bacteroides gingivalis*, *Bacteroides intermedius* and *Actinobacillus actinomycemcomitans* in human periodontal diseases. *J Clin Periodontol* **15**, 85–93.

Slots J (1982) Selective medium for isolation of *Actinobacillus actinomycetemcomitans*. *J Clin Microbiol* **15**, 606–609.

Slots J, Genco RJ (1984) Black-pigmented *Bacteroides* species, *Capnocytophaga* species and *Actinobacillus actinomycemcomitans* in human periodontal disease: virulence factors, colonization, survival and tissue destruction. *J Dent Res* **63**, 412–421.

Smaje C (1995) *Health—Race and Ethnicity*. Kings Fund Institute, London.

Smith JF (1962) Clinical evaluation of massive buccal vitamin A dosage in oral hyperkeratosis. *Oral Surgery* **15**, 282–292.

Smith CJ (1973) Global epidemiology and aetiology of oral cancer. *Cancer* **23**, 82–91.

Smith CJ (1989) Oral cancer and precancer: background, epidemiology and aetiology. *Brit Dent J* **167**, 377–383.

Smith K, Beighton D (1986) The effects of the availability of diet on the levels of exoglycosidases in the supragingival plaque of macaque monkeys. *J Dent Res* **65**, 1349–1352.

Smith DJ, Joshipura K, Kent R, Taubman MA (1992) Effects of age on immunoglobulin content and volume of human labial gland saliva. *J Dent Res* **71**, 1891–1894.

Smith AJ, Shaw L (1987) Baby fruit juices and tooth erosion. *Brit Dent J* **162**, 65–67.

Sobel AE, Saw JH, Hanok A, Nobel S (1960) Calcification XXVI: caries susceptibility in relation to composition of teeth and diet. *J Dent Res* **39**, 462–472.

Sognnaes RF, Wolcott RB, Xhonga FA (1972) Dental erosion 1: erosion-like patterns occurring in association with other dental conditions. *J Am Dent Assoc* **84**, 571–576.

Speight PM, Morgan PR (1993) The natural history and pathology of oral cancer and precancer. *Commun Dent Health* **10**s, 31–41.

Spencer N (1996) *Poverty and Child Health*. Radcliffe Medical Press, Oxford.

Spolsky VW, Atchison KA, Marcus M (1996) The dental caries experience of a Hispanic sample in Los Angeles. *J Dent Res* **75**, 186.

Spring JA, Buss DH (1977) Three centuries of alcohol in the British diet. *Nature* **270**, 567–572.

Sreebny LM (1982) Sugar availability, sugar consumption and dental caries. *Comm Dent Oral Epidemiol* **10**, 1–7.

Sreebny LM (1983) Cereal availability and dental caries. *Comm Dent Oral Epidemiol* **11**, 148–155.

Sreebny LM, Swartz SS (1997) A reference guide to drugs and dry mouth, 2nd edn. *Gerodontology* **14**, 33–48.

Staat RW, Gawronski TH, Cressy DE, Harris RS, Folke LE (1975) Effects of dietary sucrose levels on the quantity and microbial composition of human dental plaque. *J Dent Res* **54**, 872–880.

Stabholz A, Raisten J, Markitziu A *et al.* (1983) Tooth enamel dissolution from erosion or etching and subsequent caries development. *J Pedodontol* **7**, 100–108.

Stanton G (1969) Diet and Dental Caries: the phosphate sequestration hypothesis. *NY State Dent J* **35**, 399–407.

Stecksen-Blicks C (1987) Lactobacillus and *Streptococcus mutans* in saliva, diet and caries increment in 8–13-year-old children. *Scand J Dent Res* **95**, 18–26.

Steckson-Blicks C, Holm A-K (1995) Between meal eating, toothbrushing frequency and dental caries in 4-year-old children in the north of Sweden. *Int J Paediat Dent* **5**, 67–72.

Steele JG, Ayatollahi SM, Walls AW, Murray JJ (1997) Clinical factors related to reported satisfaction with oral function amongst dentate older adults in England. *Comm Dent Oral Epidemiol* **25**, 143–149.

Steele JG, Sheiham A, Marcenes W, Walls AWG (1998) *National Diet and Nutrition Survey: People aged 65 years or over*, Vol. 2: Report of the Oral Health Survey. Stationery Office, London.

Steele JG, Walls AW, Ayatollahi SM, Murray JJ (1996) Major clinical findings from a dental survey of elderly people in three different English Communities. *Brit Dent J* **180**, 17–23.

Stephan RM (1966) Effects of different types of food on dental health in experimental animals. *J Dent Res* **45**, 1551–1561.

Stephen KW, Boyle IT, Campell D, McNee S, Boyle P (1984) Five-year double-blind fluoridated milk study in Scotland. *Comm Dent Oral Epidemiol* **12**, 223–229.

Stephen KW, Banoczy J, Pakhomov GN (eds) (1996) *Milk Fluoridation for the Prevention of Dental Caries*. World Health Organisation, Geneva.

Stevens JC, Cain WS, Demarque A, Ruthruff AM (1991) On the discrimination of missing ingredients: aging and salt flavor. *Appetite* **16**, 129–140.

Stevens JC, Cain WS (1993) Changes in taste and flavor in aging. *Crit Rev Food Sci Nutr* **33**, 27–37.

Stimmler L, Snodgrass GJ, Jaffe E (1973) Dental effects associated with neonatal symptomatic hypocalcaemia. *Arch Disease Childh* **48**, 217–221.

Storkey M, Lewis R (1996) London: a true cosmopolis. In *Ethnicity in the 1991 Census*, Vol. 3 (ed P Ratcliffe). HMSO, London.

Suchman EA, Rothman A (1993) The utilisation of services. *Int Dent J* **43**, 9–16.

Summers RA, Williams SA, Curzon MEJ (1994) The use of tobacco and betel quid (pan) among Bangladeshi women in West Yorkshire. *Commun Dent Health* **11**, 12–16.

Sundby P (1967) *Alcoholism and Mortality*. National Institute for Alcohol Research, Publication No. 6, Universitetsforlaget, Oslo.

Sundqvist G (1992) Associations between microbial species in dental root canal infections. *Oral Microbiol Immunol* **7**, 257–262.

Sundqvist G, Carlsson J, Herrmann B, Tarnvik A (1985) Degradation of human immunoglobulins G and M and complement factors C3 and C5 by black pigmented Bacteroides. *J Med Microbiol* **19**, 85–94.

Sutcliffe P (1977) Caries experience and oral cleanliness of 3–4-year old children from deprived and non-deprived areas in Edinburgh, Scotland. *Comm Dent Oral Epidemiol* **5**, 213–291.

Sweeney EA, Saffir AJ, Leon R (1971) Linear enamel hypoplasia of deciduous incisor teeth in malnourished children. *Am J Clin Nutr* **24**, 29–31.

Swerdlow AJ, Marmot MG, Grulich AE, Head J (1995) Cancer mortality in Indian and British ethnic immigrants from the Indian subcontinent to England and Wales. *Brit J Canc* **72**, 1312–1319.

Szpunar SM, Eklund SA, Burt BA (1995) Sugar consumption and caries risk in schoolchildren with low caries experience. *Comm Dent Oral Epidemiol* **23**, 142–146.

Takeuchi M (1961) Epidemiological study on dental caries in Japanese children before, during and after World War II. *Int Dent J* **11**, 443–457.

Taft LI, Hughes A, Wood IJ (1958) Tongue biopsy. The technique using a rigid suction tube. *Lancet* **ii**, 69–71.

Tanner ARC (1991) Microbial succession in the development of periodontal disease. In *Periodontal Disease Pathogens and Host Immune Response* (eds S Hamada, SC Holt, JR McGhee). Quinteessence Publishing, Tokyo.

Tanzer JM (1986) Testing food cariogenicity in experimental animals. *J Dent Res* **65**, 1491–1497.

ter Steeg PF, Van der Hoeven JS, de Jong MH, van Munster PJ, Jansen M (1987) Enrichment of subgingival microflora on human serum leading to accumulation of Bacteroides species, Peptostreptococci and Fusobacteria. *Antonie Van Leeuwenhoek* **53**, 261–272.

Terpenning M, Bretz W, Lopatin D, Langmore S, Dominguez B, Loesche W (1993) Bacterial colonization of saliva and plaque in the elderly. *Clin Infect Diseases* **16**, S314–S316.

Theaker H, Porter SR (1989) Vitamin B12 deficiency and dysplasia of the oral mucosa. *Oral Surg, Oral Med, Oral Pathol* **67**, 81–83.

Thomas AK (1957) Further observations on the influence of citrus fruit juices on human teeth. *NY Soc Dent J* **23**, 424–430.

Thomas M, Avery V (1997) *Infant Feeding in Asian Families*. Office for National Statistics, London.

Thylstrup A, Fejerskov O (1978) Clinical appearance of dental fluorosis in permanent teeth in relation to histologic changes. *Comm Dent Oral Epidemiol* **6**, 315–328.

Todd JE, Dodd T (1985) *Children's Dental Health in the United Kingdom 1983*. HMSO, London.

Todd JE, Lader D (1991) *Adult Dental Health 1988 United Kingdom*. HMSO, London.

Todd JE, Walker AM (1980) *Adult Dental Health; England and Wales 1968–1978*. HMSO, London.

Toth BB, Martin JW, Lippman SM, Hong WK (1993) Chemoprevention as a form of cancer control. *J Am Dent Assoc* **124**, 243–246.

Toth K (1976) A study of 8 years' domestic salt fluoridation for prevention of caries. *Comm Dent Oral Epidemiol* **4**, 106–110.

Trowell HC, Davies JNP, Dean RFA (1952) Kwashiorkor II. Clinical picture, pathology and differential diagnosis. *Brit Med J* **2**, 798–801.

Tuyns AJ, Estere J, Raymond L *et al.* (1988) Cancer of the larynx/hypopharynx, tobacco and alcohol: IARC international study in Turin and Varese (Italy), Zaragossa and Navarra (Spain), Geneva (Switzerland) and Calvados (France). *Int J Canc* **41**, 482–491.

Tynan JJ, Kamiyama K (1984) Cystic fibrosis and oral health. *J Canadian Dent Assoc* **50**, 833–835.

US National Academy of Sciences Committee on Toxicology (1993). *Health Effects of Ingested Fluoride*. National Academy Press, Washington DC.

van der Hoeven JS, Toorop AI, Mikx RH (1978) Symbiotic relationship of *Veillonella alcalescens* and *Streptococcus mutans* in dental plaque in gnotobiotic rats. *Caries Res* **12**, 142–147.

van der Hoeven JS, van den Kieboom CW, Camp PJ (1990) Utilization of mucin by oral Streptococcus species. *Antonie Van Leeuwenhoek* **57**, 165–172.

van Houte J, Lopman J, Kent R (1994) The predominant cultivable flora of sound and carious human root surfaces. *J Dent Res* **73**, 1727–1734.

van Houte J, Lopman J, Kent R (1996) The final pH of bacteria comprising the predominant flora on sound and carious human root and enamel surfaces. *J Dent Res* **75**, 1008–1014.

van Houte J, Sansone C, Joshipura K, Kent R (1991) Mutans streptococci and non mutans streptococci acidogenic at low pH, and in vitro acidogenic potential of dental plaque in two different areas of the human dentition. *J Dent Res* **70**, 1503–1507.

van Palenstein Helderman WH, Matee MI, van der Hoeven JS, Mikx FH. (1996) Cariogenicity depends more on diet than the prevailing mutans streptococcal species. *J Dent Res* **75**, 535–545.

Van Wyk CW (1965) The oral mucosa in kwashiorkor. *J Dent Assoc South Africa* **20**, 298–302.

Van Wyk CW (1982) The etiology of oral cancer. *J Dent Assoc South Africa* **37**, 509–512.

Vandamme P, Falsen E, Rossau R *et al.* (1991) Revision of Campylobacter, Helicobacter, and Wolinella taxonomy: recomendation of generic descriptions and proposal of *Arcobacter* gen. nov. *Int J Syst Bacteriol* **41**, 88–103.

Vinson PP (1922) Hysterical dysphagia. *Minnesota Med* **5**, 107–108.

Vogel RI, Deasy M (1978) The effect of folic acid on experimentally produced gingivitis. *J Prevent Dent* **5**, 30–32.

Vogel RI, Fink R, Frank O, Baker H (1978) The effect of topic application of folic acid on gingival health. *J Oral Med* **33**, 20–22.

Von de Fehr FR, Loe H, Theilade E (1970) Experimental caries in man. *Caries Res* **4**, 131–148.

Waaler SM, Assev S, Rolla G (1985) Metabolism of xylitol in dental plaque. *Scand J Dent Res* **93**, 218–221.

Waaler SM, Assev S, Rolla G (1992) Xylitol–5-P formation by dental plaque after 12 weeks' exposure to a xylitol/sorbitol containing chewing gum. *Scand J Dent Res* **100**, 319–321.

Waerhaug J (1967) Prevalence of periodontal disease in Ceylon. *Acta Odontologica Scandinavica* **25**, 205–231.

Wahi PN (1968) The epidemiology of oral and pharyngeal cancer—A report of a study in Mainpuri district, UP, India. *WHO Bull* **38**, 495–521.

Waldenström J (1938) Iron and epithelium: some clinical observations. *Acta Medica Scandinavica* **90**, 380–397.

Waldron C, Shafer W (1975) Leukoplakia revisted: a clinicopathological study of 3,256 oral leukoplakias. *Cancer* **36**, 1386–1392.

Walls AWG (1998) Drugs and the ageing mouth. In *Drug Therapy in Old Age* (eds CF George, K Woodhouse, MJ Denham, W MacLennan). John Wiley, Chichester, 437–447.

Walsh BT, Croft CB, Katz JL (1981) Anorexia nervosa and salivary gland enlargement. *Int Psychiat Med* **11**, 255–261.

Walters CB, Sherlock JC, Evans WH, Read I (1983) Dietary intake of fluoride in the United Kingdom and fluoride content of some foodstuffs. *J Sci Food Agric* **34**, 523–528.

Warnakulasuriya KAAS (1992) Smoking and chewing habits in Sri Lanka: Implications for oral cancer and precancer. In *Control of Tobacco Related Cancer and Other Diseases* (eds PC Gupta, JE Hamner II, PR Murti). Oxford University Press, Bombay, 25–46.

Warnakulasuriya KAAS (1996) Ethnicity, race and oral cancer. In *Dentists, Patients and Ethnic Minorities—Towards the New Millennium* (eds R Bedi, V Bahal, RR Rayan). The Department of Health, London.

Warnakulasuriya KAAS, Prabhu SR (1992) Anaemia in

the tropics. In *Oral Diseases in the Tropics* (eds SR Prabhu, DS Wilson, DK Daftary, NW Johnson). Oxford University Press, Oxford, 325–339.

Warnes T (1996) The age structure and ageing of the ethnic groups. In *Ethnicity in the 1991 Census*, Vol. 3 (ed P Ratcliffe). HMSO, London.

Waterlow J (1992) *Protein Energy Malnutrition*. Edward Arnold, London.

Weerheijm KL, Kidd EA, Groen HJ (1997) The effect of fluoridation on the occurrence of hidden caries in clinically sound occlusal surfaces. *Caries Res* **31**, 30–34.

Weiffenbach JM (1987) Taste perception mechanisms. In *The Aging Mouth*, Vol. 6 (ed DB Ferguson). Karger, Basle, 151–167.

Wennerholm K, Birkhed D, Emilson CG (1995) Effects of sugar restriction on *Streptococcus mutans* and *Streptococcus sobrinus* in saliva and dental palque. *Caries Res* **29**, 54–61.

Wharton P, Wharton B (1984) Nutrition of Asian children: foetus and newborn. In *Ethnic Factors in Health and Disease* (eds JK Cruickshank, DG Beevers). Wright, London.

Whiley RA, Fraser H, Hardie JM, Beighton D (1990) Phenotypic differentiation of *Streptococcus intermedius*, *Streptococcus constellatus* and *Streptococcus anginosus* (the *Streptococcus milleri* group): association with different body sites and clinical infections. *J Clin Microbiol* **28**, 1497–1501.

White A, Nicolaus G, Foster K *et al.* (1993) *Health Survey for England 1991*. HMSO, London.

White D, Anderson RJ (1996) Children's dental health under the capitation scheme. *Commun Dent Health* **13**, 21–48.

World Health Organization (WHO) (1977). *Manual of the International Statistical Classification of Diseases, Injuries, and Causes of Death* (based on the recommendations of the ninth revision conference). WHO, Geneva.

WHO (1994) *Fluorides and Oral Health*. WHO, Geneva.

WHO (1989) *A Review of Current Recommendations for the Organization and Administration of Community Health Services in Northern and Western Europe*. WHO Regional Office for Europe, Copenhagen.

Williams DM, Hughes FJ, Odell EW, Farthing PM (1992) *Pathology of Periodontal Disease*. Oxford University Press, Oxford.

Winn DM, Brunelle JA, Selwitz RH *et al.* (1996). Coronal and root caries in the dentition of adults in the United States. *J Dent Res* **75**, 642–651.

Winn DM, Zeigler RG, Pickle LW *et al.* (1984) Diet in the etiology of oral and pharyngeal cancer among women from the southern United States. *Cancer Res* **44**, 1216–1222.

Winter GB (1976) Maternal nutritional requirements in relation to the subsequent development of teeth in children. *J Hum Nutr* **30**, 93–99.

Winter GB (1980) Problems involved with the use of comforters. *Int Dent J* **30**, 28–38.

Winter GB (1996) Amelogenesis imperfecta with enamel opacities and taurodontism: an alternative diagnosis for 'idiopathic dental fluorosis'. *Brit Dent J* **181**, 167–172.

Woodward M, Walker AR (1994) Sugar consumption and dental caries: evidence from 90 countries. *Brit Dent J* **176**, 297–302.

Wray D (1982) A double-blind trial of systemic zinc sulphate in recurrent aphthous stomatitis. *Oral Surg, Oral Med, Oral Pathol* **53**, 469–472.

Wray D, Dagg JH (1990) Oral manifestations of diseases of the blood and blood forming organs. In *Oral Manifestations of Systemic Disease* (eds JH Jones, DK Mason), Baillière Tindall, London, 60–713.

Wray D, Ferguson MM, Hutcheon AW, Dagg JH (1978) Nutritional deficiences in recurrent aphthae. *J Oral Pathol* **7**, 418–423.

Wray D, Ferguson MM, Mason DK, Hutcheon AW, Dagg JH (1975) Recurrent aphthae: treatment with vitamin B12, folic acid and iron. *Brit Med J* **ii**, 490–493.

Wynder EL, Bross IJ, Feldman RM (1957) A study of the etiologic factors in cancer of the mouth. *Cancer* **10**, 1300–1323.

Wynder EL, Fryer JH (1958) Etiologic considerations of Plummer-Vinson (Paterson-Kelly) syndrome. *Ann Int Med* **49**, 1106–1128.

Xhonga FA, Valdmanis S (1983) Geographic comparisons of the incidence of dental erosion: a two-centre study. *J Oral Rehab* **10**, 269–277.

Young TB, Ford CN, Brandenburg JH (1986) An epidemiologic study of oral cancer in a statewide network. *Am J Orolaryngol* **7**, 200–208.

Zero DT (1996) Etiology of dental erosion—extrinsic factors. *Eur J Oral Sci* **104**, 162–177.

Zhang KH, Yu SF, Tang JQ (1995) An epidemiological survey of oral submucous fibrosis in Xiangtan City, Hunan Province, China. Proceedings of the 4th ICOOC, Gifu, Japan.

Zheng T, Boyle P, Hu H *et al.* (1990a). Tobacco smoking, alcohol consumption and risk of oral cancer: a case-control study in Beijing, People's Republic of China. *Canc Causes Control* **1**, 173–179.

Zheng T, Boyle P, Huanfang H *et al.* (1990b) Dentition, oral hygiene and risk of oral cancer: a case-control study in Beijing, People's Republic of China. *Canc Causes Control* **1**, 235–241.

Zheng T, Boyle P, Willett WC *et al.* (1993) A case-control study of oral cancer in Beijing, People's Republic of China. Associations with nutrient intakes, foods and food groups. *Eur J Canc* **29B**, 45–55.

AUTHOR INDEX

SUBJECT INDEX